The British Medical Association

FAMILY DOCTOR GUIDE *to*

PARKINSON'S DISEASE

DK The British Medical Association

FAMILY DOCTOR GUIDE *to*

PARKINSON'S DISEASE

DR. JOHN M. S. PEARCE

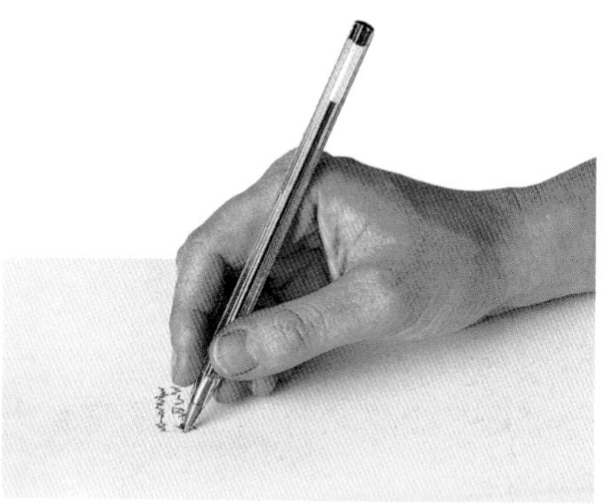

MEDICAL EDITOR
DR. TONY SMITH

DORLING KINDERSLEY
LONDON • NEW YORK • SYDNEY • MOSCOW
www.dk.com

IMPORTANT

This book is not designed as a substitute for personal medical advice but as a supplement to that advice for the patient who wishes to understand more about his/her condition.

Before taking any form of treatment **YOU SHOULD ALWAYS CONSULT YOUR MEDICAL PRACTITIONER.**

In particular (without limit) you should note that advances in medical science occur rapidly and some of the information contained in this book about drugs and treatment may very soon be out of date.

PLEASE NOTE
The author regrets that he cannot enter into any correspondence with readers.

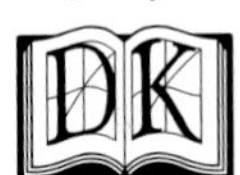

A DORLING KINDERSLEY BOOK
www.dk.com

Senior Editor Mary Lindsay
Senior Designer Sarah Hall
Production Controller Michelle Thomas

Managing Editor Stephanie Jackson
Managing Art Editor Nigel Duffield

Produced for Dorling Kindersley Limited by
Design Revolution, Queens Park Villa,
30 West Drive, Brighton, East Sussex BN2 2GE
Editorial Director Ian Whitelaw
Art Director Fiona Roberts
Editor Julie Whitaker
Designer Vanessa Good

Published in Great Britain in 1999 by
Dorling Kindersley Limited,
9 Henrietta Street, London WC2E 8PS

2 4 6 8 10 9 7 5 3 1

A CIP catalogue record for this book is available from the British Library

ISBN 07513 0671 1

Reproduced by Colourscan, Singapore
Printed in Hong Kong by Wing King Tong

Contents

Introduction

If you, or a close relative or friend, suffer from Parkinson's disease, this book is written for you. It is aimed to help you to understand the symptoms and disabilities caused by the disease and to suggest what you can do for yourself as well as what doctors can do to treat the condition.

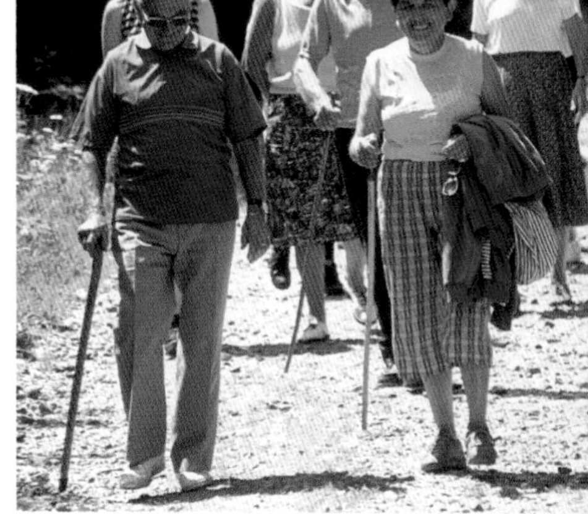

AN IMPROVED OUTLOOK
Modern treatments mean that people with Parkinson's disease can now enjoy a much more active life than sufferers in previous decades.

The good news is that, although there is still much to be learned about Parkinson's disease, the grim prospects that prevailed 30 years ago have been much improved by increased understanding and modern forms of treatment.

WHAT IS PARKINSON'S DISEASE?

Parkinson's disease is characterised by a collection of signs involving the nervous system, the most important of which are:

- Slowness of movement.
- Rigidity – the limbs may feel heavy and stiff.
- Shaking of the hands and sometimes legs at rest.
- Disorders of posture – the patient's neck and trunk assume a bent position, and the arms fail to swing freely when walking.

The disease is caused by degeneration of pigmented nerve cells in the brain. It usually starts in the 50s or 60s and can remain stationary for months or years, but usually progresses.

Parkinson's disease seldom shortens life expectancy to any significant degree.

In the advanced stages, tremor, slowness and rigidity may affect all four limbs and the trunk; speech may be indistinct and slurred, the limbs and body are bent and the victim is prone to walk with short, stumbling steps and is prone to fall.

WHO GETS IT?

Parkinson's disease may afflict people from all classes of society, from all races, and occurs throughout the world.

It increases with ageing, but is not caused by ageing itself. Overall, about one person in 1,000 is affected, but this increases to about one in 100 people in their 70s and 80s.

Many elderly people are so mildly affected by Parkinson's disease that the condition is easily overlooked.

Men and women are equally affected by Parkinson's disease, and the disease is seldom inherited.

DON'T GET TOO DEPRESSED

If this description sounds depressing, remember that for many years the disability is mild, and during this time most patients are capable of normal domestic activities and can usually maintain their normal jobs.

Furthermore, although there is no cure for Parkinson's disease at the present time, many of the symptoms can be well controlled by appropriate treatment.

HOW IS THE DIAGNOSIS MADE?

People wonder how the diagnosis is made. It is invariably a clinical decision, based on the symptoms and especially the signs that the experienced doctor can observe during an examination.

Laboratory tests and X-rays are generally unnecessary, and special tests such as computed tomography (CT) scans and magnetic resonance imaging (MRI) scans are generally unhelpful; indeed such scans often give a normal result in Parkinson's disease.

HOW IS IT TREATED ?

Treatment is based on the replacement of those chemicals in the brain that are reduced or depleted by Parkinson's disease. The main chemical to be affected by Parkinson's disease is dopamine, which diminishes slowly for a number of years before any symptoms become apparent.

It is estimated that you have to lose 80 per cent of the dopamine in the critical areas of your brain before symptoms or signs are evident. Dopamine is found in groups of nerve cells in the base of the brain, called the basal ganglia.

Patients are given a drug called levodopa to replace the missing dopamine, but other drugs are used too.

Physiotherapy, speech and occupational therapy can all be valuable physical therapies at certain stages for patients with Parkinson's disease. These supplement, but are not an effective substitute for, drug treatment. The aim throughout treatment is to maintain your activity and allow you to follow as near-normal a lifestyle as possible.

WHO WILL TREAT YOU?

Patients and their families have to be as active as the doctors and therapists. Your GP will be the first person to consult, and indeed may assume responsibility for managing your condition, including making the diagnosis, explaining and prescribing drugs and possibly organising physiotherapy and occupational therapy. The GP may then refer you to a consultant, ideally a neurologist, although it could be a general physician or a geriatrician. The consultant will write to your own GP confirming the diagnosis and advising him or her about treatment.

Once the diagnosis has been confirmed and treatment started, the GP will provide continuing care, although he or she will probably refer you back to the consultant if any problems arise.

KEY POINTS

- Parkinson's disease can affect people from all races and social classes, and men and women are equally affected.
- The illness is most common in elderly people.
- Symptoms can be controlled by appropriate treatment.

Causes and characteristics

The essential cause is not known. Clues are available from studies of the distribution of the disease – that is, who is affected, where and in what circumstances. I have already mentioned that it is relatively common – perhaps as many as 100,000 patients are affected in the UK at any one time – that men and women are equally affected, and that no race is immune.

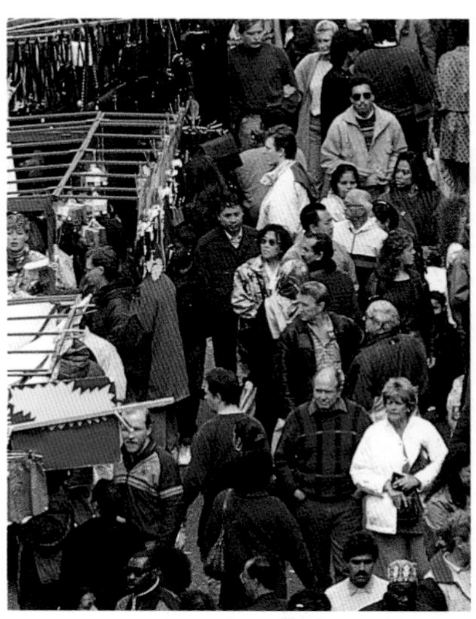

DEMOCRATIC DISEASE
Parkinson's disease is equally common among men and women, and does not affect one occupation or ethnic group more than another.

Parkinson's disease is not related to any particular job and is clearly a physical disease of the brain, which is not caused by stress, anxiety or family upsets. Extensive searches for a viral or bacterial cause have proved negative, so the disease is not infectious.

NERVE CELL DEGENERATION

In patients with Parkinson's disease, there is disease or degeneration of the so-called basal ganglia in the deeper grey matter of the brain, particularly of that part known as the substantia nigra.

The Function of the Substantia Nigra

Nerve cells in the substantia nigra, in the upper part of the brain stem, contain the neurotransmitter dopamine. Nerve fibres in these cells release dopamine into the corpus striatum, a part of the brain that controls movement.

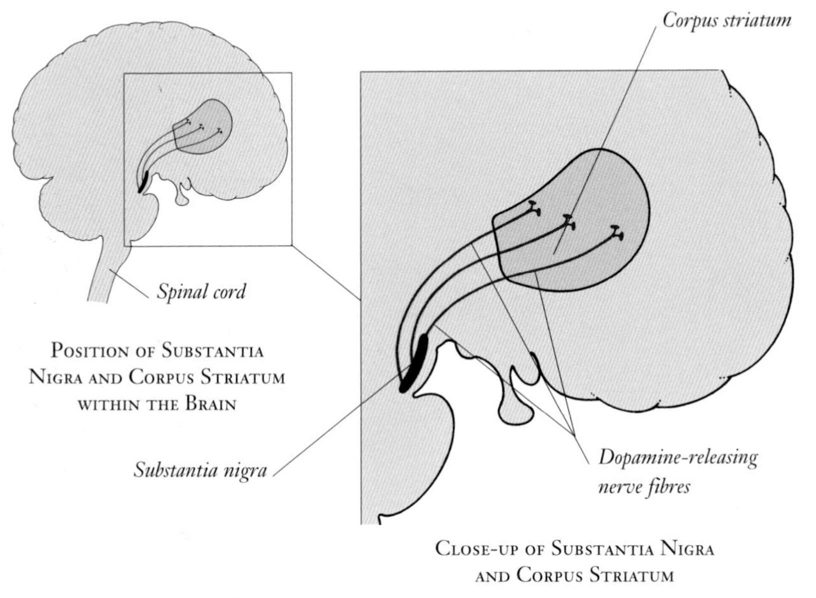

POSITION OF SUBSTANTIA NIGRA AND CORPUS STRIATUM WITHIN THE BRAIN

CLOSE-UP OF SUBSTANTIA NIGRA AND CORPUS STRIATUM

The substantia nigra, which connects with the striatum (caudate nucleus and globus pallidus), contains black pigmented cells and, in normal individuals, produces a number of chemical transmitters, the most important of which is dopamine. Other transmitters include serotonin, somatostatin and noradrenaline. With Parkinson's disease, the basal ganglia cells produce less dopamine, which is needed to transmit vital messages to other parts of the brain, and to the spinal cord, nerves and muscles.

The basal ganglia, through the action of dopamine, are responsible for planning and controlling automatic movements of the body, such as pointing with a finger, pulling on a sock, writing or walking. If the basal ganglia are not working properly, as in Parkinson's disease patients, all aspects of movement are impaired, resulting in the characteristic features of the disease – slowness of movement, stiffness and effort required to move a limb and, often, tremor.

Dopamine levels in the brain's substantia nigra do normally fall with ageing. However, they have to fall to one-fifth of normal values for the symptoms and signs of parkinsonism to emerge.

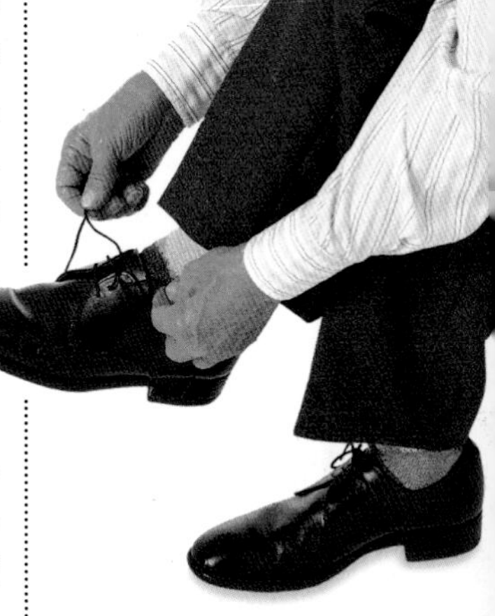

PRACTICAL PROBLEMS
People with Parkinson's disease find their movements become slow and stiff, and they have problems with semi-automatic tasks such as tying shoelaces.

RESTORING THE BALANCE

Normally, there is a balance between dopamine and another neurotransmitter, which is called acetylcholine.

How Drug Treatment Works

Brain cell degeneration in Parkinson's disease cannot be stopped, but drugs can minimise the effects for years. They help to restore the balance between dopamine and acetylcholine by boosting dopamine levels and inactivating some acetylcholine.

Imbalanced state with relative excess acetylcholine

Dopamine

BEFORE DRUG TREATMENT

Acetylcholine inactivated by drug

Dopamine plus levodopa

Balanced state

Dopamine

Active acetylcholine

AFTER DRUG TREATMENT

Acetylcholine is present in many areas of the brain and plays a part in normal memory recording and recall. Because dopamine is depleted, there is a relative excess of acetylcholine. Thus, two of the main groups of drugs used to treat Parkinson's disease are dopamine drugs (levodopa and its preparations Madopar and Sinemet) and drugs designed to restore the balance by diminishing the acetylcholine – anticholinergics (for example, Artane, Disipal, Cogentin).

HOW DO NERVE CELLS SEND MESSAGES?

The diagram opposite shows how a nerve cell, or neurone, in the basal ganglia transmits a nerve impulse down its main wire, or axon, to the synaptic knob, which releases a package of dopamine. When this passes into receptors of the next nerve cell, it transmits the message further down the line. You can imagine this process carried out by millions of neurones at the same time, forming a network of activity that puts BT to shame.

Current ideas about the cause of Parkinson's disease suggest that some people are born with a predisposition that makes them vulnerable to some (unidentified) environmental toxic agents. Why cells die in the substantia nigra of Parkinson's disease patients is unknown. This important group of cells shows three changes:

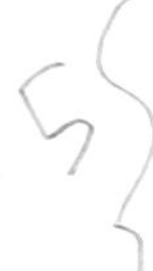

- Evidence of the release of oxygen compound by cells which act as a stress that damages cells (oxidative stress), and depletion of a chemical called reduced glutathione.
- High levels of iron.
- A deficiency of an essential component of all cells (mitochondrial complex 1) that normally controls oxidative reactions.

How Dopamine Conducts Nerve Impulses

When electrical impulses passing along the axon of a nerve cell reach the synaptic knob, stored dopamine is released. This passes across the gap, or synapse, to receptors in the next nerve cell, causing an impulse to pass along the second cell.

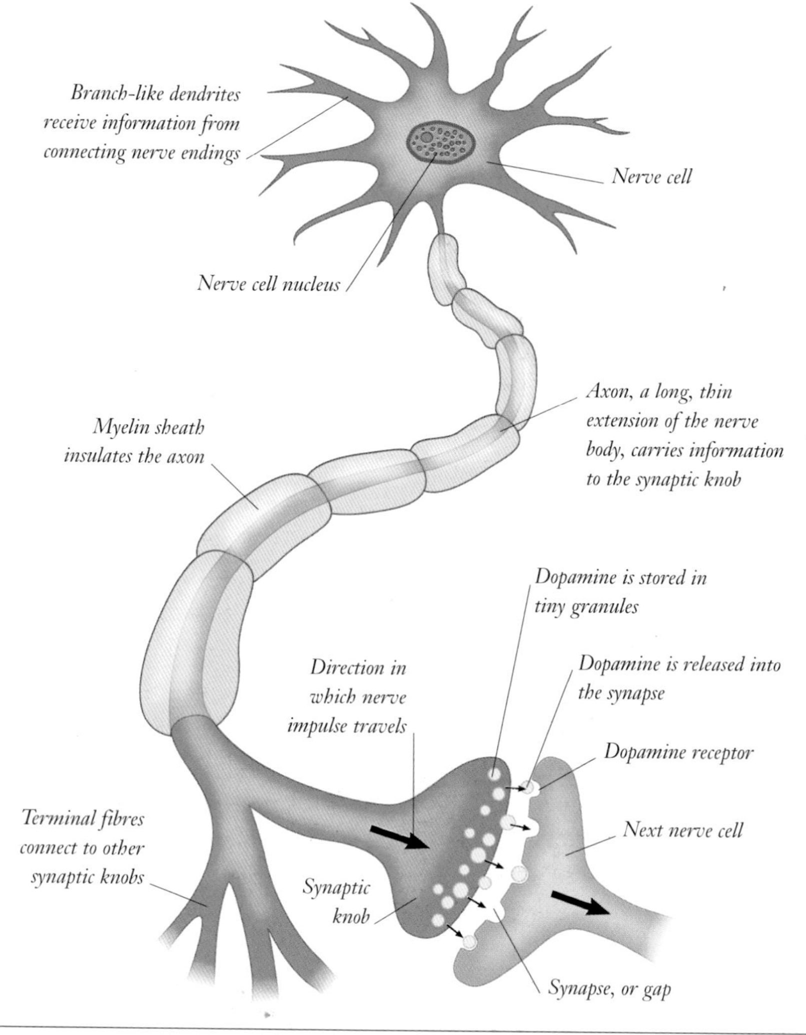

Which of these is the primary event, causing secondary changes culminating in substantia nigral cell death, is not known. In presymptomatic subjects with Lewy bodies in their brains, the substantia nigra shows a comparable loss of reduced glutathione and, possibly, a reduction of complex 1 activity. These various abnormalities provide a new focus for the development of future treatments.

The receptors are most important. Some drugs can block the receptors, and if they are taken for a long period they block the passage of dopamine in the nerve cells and their connecting network of axons. The nerve impulses, so essential for normal movement, are therefore reduced. This is the basis of the drug-induced parkinsonism I shall describe in the next chapter.

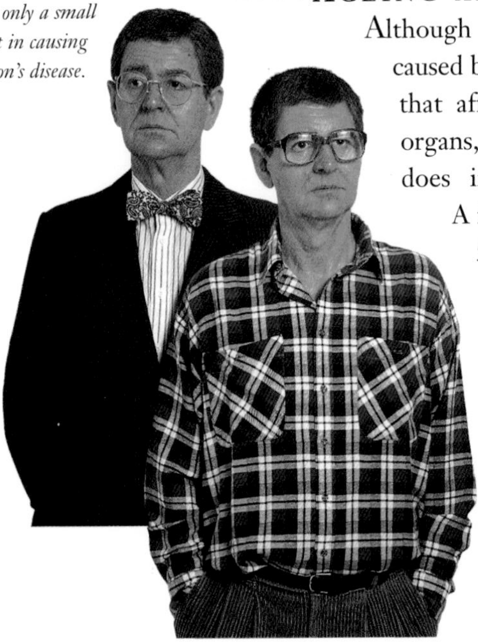

Twin Studies
Studies of twins suggest that hereditary factors play only a small part in causing Parkinson's disease.

Ageing and Heredity

Although Parkinson's disease is not caused by the normal ageing process that affects our brains and other organs, the incidence of the disease does increase as we get older. A family history is obtained in 5–10 per cent of patients, but studies that have been made on twins suggest that hereditary factors are relatively unimportant. It may prove to be that affected relatives share some unknown environmental agent, or that they are genetically vulnerable to it.

KEY POINTS

- The cause of Parkinson's disease is unknown.
- Research has shown that pigment-containing cells in the deep part of the brain that produce dopamine and other important chemicals degenerate and die. This, in turn, affects the working of other parts of the brain, the spinal cord, nerves and muscles involved in movement.
- When the chemical dopamine is depleted, there is a relative excess of the chemical acetylcholine.
- Treatment is aimed at boosting dopamine levels and/or diminishing acetylcholine levels.

Types of parkinsonism

We separate Parkinson's disease (idiopathic Parkinson's disease or paralysis agitans), described by James Parkinson in 1817, from a group of rarer disorders also caused by impairment of the function of the nerve cells of the brain, and called secondary or symptomatic parkinsonism.

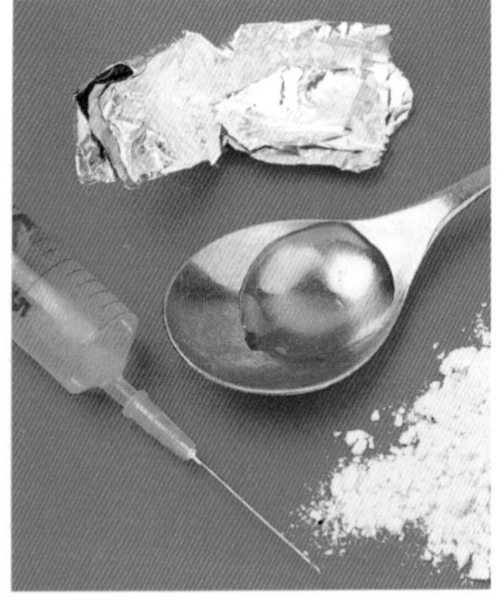

AN EFFECT OF DRUG ABUSE
A chemical that is found in drugs used by heroin addicts has been found to cause symptomatic parkinsonism very quickly.

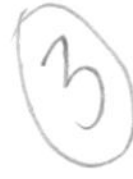

There are several kinds of symptomatic parkinsonism:

- Drug-induced parkinsonism.
- So-called post-encephalitic parkinsonism.
- Poison-induced parkinsonism.
- Multiple system atrophies.

It is important to distinguish between true Parkinson's disease and symptomatic parkinsonism, because the treatment may be quite different.

DRUG-INDUCED

Neuroleptic drugs used in the treatment of schizophrenia and other serious psychotic mental illnesses, can block the release or transmission of dopamine in the substantia nigra and striatum, causing parkinsonism. The most common neuroleptic drugs are the phenothiazines, but there are many others, as shown in the table on p.20. The list is not complete, and if in doubt, you should ask your GP or consultant whether the drug you are taking might cause parkinsonism.

Some of these drugs are used to counter nausea, vomiting or dizziness and, under these circumstances, parkinsonism should not develop if the course of treatment is restricted to less than a month. If it is possible for your physician to withdraw the drugs, the parkinsonism will usually slowly disappear, though this may take several months. Some patients with serious psychiatric illness need to continue the neuroleptic drugs; some degree of parkinsonism then has to be tolerated to maintain mental stability, and can usually be controlled.

POST-ENCEPHALITIC

This type of parkinsonism is now extremely rare. It developed in the wake of a diffuse inflammation of the brain (encephalitis) caused by an epidemic of a particular virus infection that raged throughout the world between 1918 and 1926. The symptoms and treatment are slightly different from those of idiopathic Parkinson's disease.

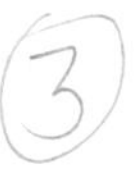

POISON-INDUCED

It has been found that MPTP, a chemical contaminant of do-it-yourself drugs made illegally and used by heroin addicts, mainly in California, can produce parkinsonism within days or weeks. The brains in fatal cases show severe destruction of the substantia nigra, and profound loss of dopamine and other neural transmitters, as is seen in Parkinson's disease.

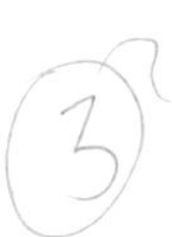

Their symptoms are controlled by levodopa drugs, which replace the missing dopamine in just the same way as in Parkinson's disease. However, the brain damage inflicted by MPTP is permanent. Researchers now have

Drugs that Can Cause Parkinsonism

Below is a list of neuroleptic drugs – used in the treatment of serious psychiatric illnesses such as schizophrenia – that have been known to cause symptomatic parkinsonism.

COMMONLY USED NEUROLEPTIC DRUGS	SIMILAR NEUROLEPTIC ANTIPSYCHOTIC DRUGS	NEUROLEPTIC DRUGS GIVEN BY INJECTION
Chlorpromazine (Largactil)	Benperidol (Anquill)	Flupenthixol (Depixol)
Fluphenazine (Moditen, Motival)	Droperiodol (Droleptan)	Fluphenazine (Modecate, Moditen)
Promazine (Sparine)	Flupenthixol (Depixol, Fluanxol)	Fluspirilene (Redeptin)
Trifluoperazine (Stelazine)	Zuclopenthixol (Clopixol)	Haloperidol (Haldol)
Prochlorperazine (Stemetil)	Haloperidol (Serenace, Haldol, Dozic)	Pipothiazine (Piportil)
Thioridazine (Melleril)	Reserpine (Serpasil, Decaserpyl)	
Pericyazine (Neulactil)	Tetrabenazine (Nitoman)	
Perphenazine (Fentazin, Triptafen)	Sulpiride (Dolmatil)	
	Pimozide (Orap)	
	Risperidone (Risperdal)	

proof that certain poisons can damage the brain in a way similar to that arising spontaneously in idiopathic Parkinson's disease – a valuable finding for further research into the sequence of events leading to degeneration of the dopamine-generating cells. For example, in animal experiments in which parkinsonism is artificially induced using MPTP, it has been shown that the dopamine-producing cells in the substantia nigra are deficient in one of the important enzymes known as complex-1, involved in oxygen control in the cell. In spite of improved knowledge and understanding of the nature and causes of Parkinson's disease, more work needs to be done to further our knowledge and to develop better treatment.

OTHER TYPES

Parkinsonism is not normally a feature of head injury and is seldom a symptom of a brain tumour. Other disorders, characterised by rigid akinetic states can result from a variety of other degenerations of the brain, including the conditions known as progressive supranuclear palsy, multisystem atrophies and Lewy body disease. All these conditions are rare causes of parkinsonism and require specialised neurological assessment; they do not all respond well to anti-parkinsonian drugs.

KEY POINT

- Parkinson's disease needs to be distinguished from various types of symptomatic parkinsonism because the treatment may be different.

Symptoms and signs

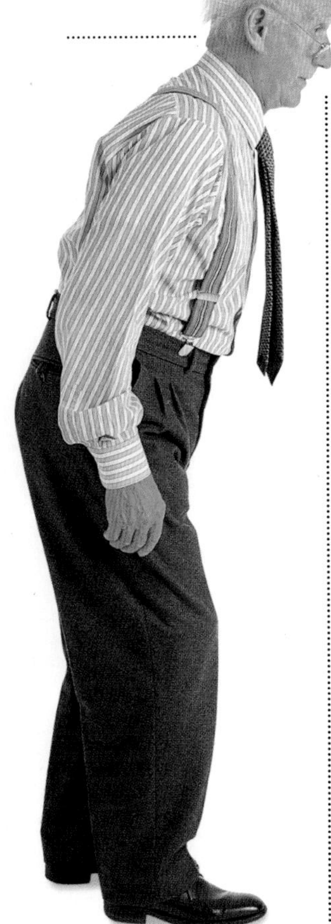

COMMON SYMPTOM
Patients often tend to lean forwards from their centre of gravity when they walk.

As I have mentioned earlier, the principal physical symptoms that affect people suffering from Parkinson's disease are tremor, muscular rigidity, akinesia, abnormal posture and loss of balance.

WHAT ARE THE SYMPTOMS?

Let's look at these symptoms in more detail, bearing in mind that different patients will experience symptoms to varying degrees.

TREMOR

The commonest early symptom is shaking (tremor) of one or both hands. It occurs at rest, and is reduced or stopped when the limb is in action. It is fairly slow – about five beats per second, and rhythmical. It usually vanishes during sleep.

RIGIDITY

Rigidity means stiffness and a sense of effort required to move the limb, which may feel heavy and weak. However, loss of strength and power is not a feature of Parkinson's disease.

SLOW MOVEMENT

Slowness of movement can be experienced in three ways: lack of spontaneous movement (akinesia), slowness in starting a movement, and slowness during the movement itself (bradykinesia). The patient's handwriting tends to become progressively smaller (called micrographia, from Latin *micro*: small, and *graphos:* writing) and the writing may show signs of the tremor.

DISORDERS OF POSTURE

Disorders of posture is the term that refers to the bent position of the neck and trunk that develops late in the disease. It describes the way the arms are held close to the sides, elbows and wrists slightly bent; the legs, too, may be flexed at the hips and knees.

Common Symptoms of Parkinson's Disease

Although the symptoms of Parkinson's disease vary from patient to patient, there is a range of common shared characteristics.

- Difficulty fastening buttons
- Inability to turn over
- Inability to get up from the chair
- Expressionless face
- Falls frequently
- Feet freeze
- Greasy skin
- Rarely blinks
- Shuffling steps
- Slow eating
- Slow movement
- Soft voice
- Stiff limbs
- Tremor

LOSS OF BALANCE

Loss of balance often accompanies disordered posture. Patients find it difficult to correct a trip or stumble (lack of righting reflexes) and, as a consequence, are prone to fall. They seem to lean forwards in front of their centre of gravity and, without being able to help themselves, a walk may break into a run (called festination by doctors, from the Latin *festinare*: to hurry). Or, if pushed gently, patients may uncontrollably run forwards or stumble backwards.

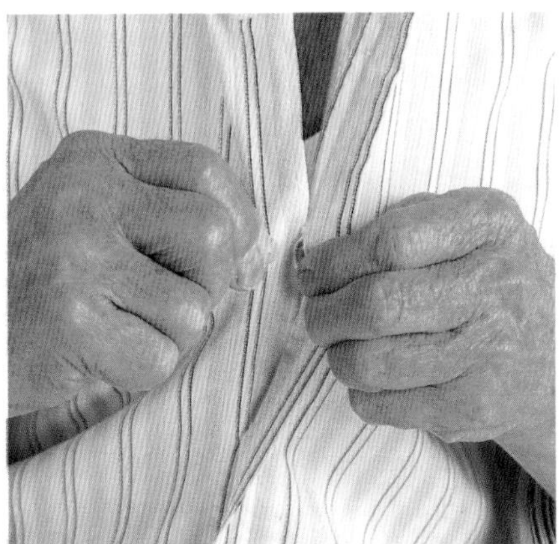

DRESSING DIFFICULTIES
Stiffness and slowness of movement can cause difficulty in fastening buttons, making everyday dressing frustrating.

SIGNS

When your doctor examines, you he will notice certain signs, though as with the symptoms, these vary from patient to patient, and change in the individual at different times. For example, your movements may be visibly slow (bradykinesia: *brady* – slow, *kinesis* – movement). You may rise slowly from the chair, or walk slowly with short steps into the consulting room. You may have a slow rhythmic tremor of one or both arms that disappears on grasping a chair or taking hold of an object. Many years ago, this was likened to rolling pills made by hand: pill-rolling tremor. When the doctor bends or straightens your wrist or arm or legs he may feel a sense of resistance like trying to bend a lead pipe; he may also feel the tremor superimposed, creating a sensation of turning a cogwheel (known as cogwheel rigidity).

AUTOMATIC MOVEMENTS

Actions are noticeably laboured. Most of us perform automatic movements unconsciously at rest, when sitting comfortably. Such movements – blinking, crossing and uncrossing the legs and general fidgeting, for example – are lacking in the Parkinson's disease patient. When walking, Parkinson's disease patients use short steps and shuffle, as if the feet are glued to the floor. Gait is hesitant, and steps shorten even more in doorways, or when there is an obstruction, or, if in the street, a passing dog or a stranger runs across their path. Sometimes patients get stuck when walking; their feet feel frozen to the ground. If this happens to you, deliberately focus on a spot in front of you and aim at it with the leading leg: you will find you can usually start to walk again.

FACIAL APPEARANCE AND SPEECH

The face may lack expression, the eyes are a little staring, and in advanced cases, there is a tendency to dribble saliva. This arises, not because of excessive formation, but because of reduction in the normal swallowing of saliva that we do unconsciously and automatically. The voice is quiet, sometimes hoarse (dysphonia), and the words may be slurred (dysarthria). These problems may be inconspicuous, but may manifest themselves as difficulty singing in the bath or, more embarrassingly, in the choir.

CHANGED BLADDER AND BOWEL HABITS

Constipation is almost invariable. It is caused by sluggish movement of the muscle in the bowel, very similar to that seen in the limbs. It is not a serious symptom, but it does cause much concern and apprehension, particularly in the elderly.

The bladder muscle, too, contracts less efficiently, and frequent calls to pass urine are common, with small volumes and some measure of urgency. In older men, coincidental enlargement of the prostate may add to the problems, with a slow stream and the need to get up at night to pass urine.

If you suffer from these problems, you may need to be assessed by both a neurologist and a urologist. Incontinence does not occur in the early stages of the illness, and if it does occur later, it may have some other explanation. You may have accidents because of physical slowness, being unable to get to the toilet in time; this is not true incontinence but urgency incontinence, and this can sometimes be improved by treatment with drugs such as oxybutynin.

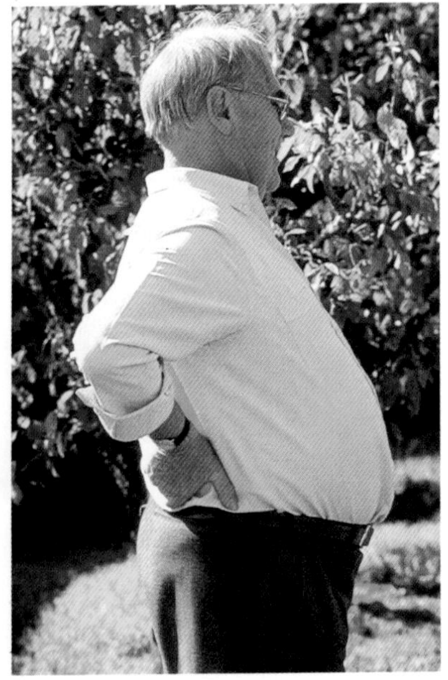

STIFFNESS IN THE BACK *Sufferers sometimes experience aching and stiffness in the back, neck and limbs, making movement difficult.*

SWALLOWING DIFFICULTIES

Occasionally, difficulty in swallowing develops as a result of the Parkinson's disease, but special tests are needed to make sure this symptom is not due to causes other than parkinsonism, which may have arisen by chance.

OTHER PROBLEMS

Usually, these are late features that appear after many years of illness. Most patients are able to walk well, to speak clearly and to work and enjoy leisure activities for many years. Modern specialist treatment by a neurologist can control symptoms effectively in most sufferers.

Other problems occasionally trouble patients. Pain is not a serious problem for most sufferers, though aching and stiffness in the neck, back and limbs is quite common. Because of reduced automatic movement, a stiff or frozen shoulder may develop. This is painful and stops men getting to their wallets in their back trouser pockets, and causes women difficulties with zips and bra fasteners. These incidental problems can be treated effectively.

Occasionally, patients are affected by writer's cramp. Drug side-effects can also cause symptoms.

KEY POINTS

- Symptoms of Parkinson's disease include tremor, rigidity, akinesia, disorders of posture and loss of balance.
- Symptoms vary a great deal, and later in the illness may include changed bladder and bowel habits, and difficulty in swallowing.
- Signs include reduced automatic movements, altered facial appearance and speech.

How is the diagnosis made?

Some patients, and even more of their relations, worry about the accuracy of the diagnosis. One patient differs from the next, and your symptoms and your appearance may be different from those of the chap shaking away in your local or in the corner shop, who is said to have Parkinson's disease. In most cases an accurate diagnosis is not difficult.

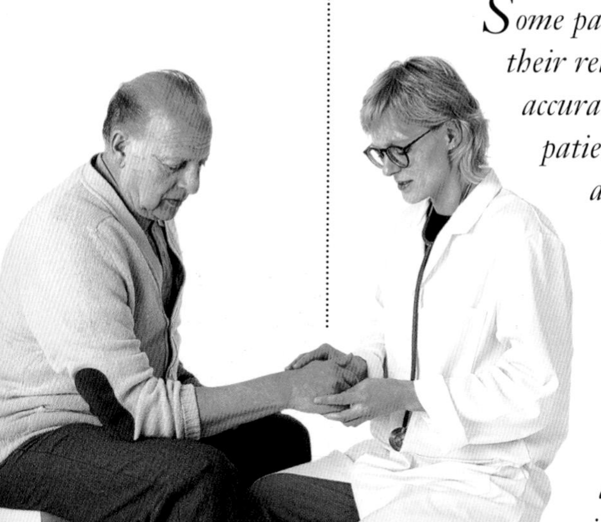

MAKING A DIAGNOSIS
Although there are no clinical tests to confirm a diagnosis, the signs and symptoms of Parkinson's disease are usually easy to detect with an expert eye.

As with certain other diseases, there are no specific or diagnostic tests that confirm or refute a diagnosis of Parkinson's disease. Blood tests, electroencephalograms (EEG), computed tomography (CT) and magnetic resonance imaging (MRI) scans are essentially normal.

Parkinson's disease can be mistaken for other diseases, and since the outlook and treatment may be substantially different, it is generally advisable for the initial suspicion to be confirmed or rejected by a consultant neurologist.

The diagnosis is based on the history and signs, and to the expert eye, may be immediately evident when the patient enters the consulting room. A change in handwriting, dragging of one leg without hip disease or a complaint of clumsiness will all alert the doctor to the possible diagnosis. The severity and the type of illness will be explored in this clinical examination and the disability will be shown by questioning about what you can and cannot do.

DISEASES WITH SIMILAR SIGNS

You can see from the tables on p.30 that there are other causes of shaking and tremors that can be mistaken for Parkinson's disease.

The most frequent is a common, fairly harmless condition called benign essential tremor, which occurs in 2–4 per cent of the population, in varying degree. Here, the shaking is slight or absent at rest, but worse when the arms are held stretched out; there is usually no rigidity or slowness of movement, and no tendency to a bent or flexed posture. It often, but not always, runs in families, and the tremor may be reduced by a small dose of alcohol. This condition does not respond to anti-parkinsonian drugs.

Thyroid disease, alcoholism, anxiety states and a variety of rare metabolic and structural disorders can occasionally mimic Parkinson's disease, but these will be suspected by the specialist if the symptoms are unusual, and it is only then that investigations may be suggested. These conditions are rarely a diagnostic problem, so tests are not undertaken in most patients.

SHARED SYMPTOM
Diseases such as benign essential tremor can also cause handwriting to become shaky, but with Parkinson's disease the writing also becomes smaller.

Conditions with Symptoms that Look Like Parkinson's Disease

A number of neurological diseases produce physical symptoms that may mimic Parkinson's disease.

- Post-encephalitic parkinsonism; drug-induced parkinsons.
- Other causes of tremor – such as benign essential tremor, thyrotoxicosis or alcoholism
- Other brain disease – such as multiple strokes

Diseases that People Commonly Confuse with Parkinson's Disease

Parkinson's disease is sometimes confused with other, unrelated conditions, some of which can produce similar symptoms.

- Brain tumour
- Strokes
- Multiple sclerosis
- After-effects of head injury
- Alzheimer's disease and primary dementias
- Motor neurone disease

MULTIPLE SCLEROSIS AND STROKES

Occasionally, people who are subsequently diagnosed as having Parkinson's disease wonder if it is multiple sclerosis, or some form of unusual stroke. Multiple sclerosis is mainly a disease of younger people, and its symptoms and signs are quite different and will be quickly appreciated by the specialist.

Multiple strokes affecting in turn each side of the body can, rarely, produce a picture that superficially resembles

Parkinson's disease; here, expert opinion will separate the two conditions. Of course, both conditions can arise by chance in the same unfortunate individual, but the specialist will usually be able to clarify the issue. Strokes do not, however, cause Parkinson's disease.

ALZHEIMER'S DISEASE

Sometimes the more advanced or elderly patient may suffer from loss of memory, or develop periods of confusion. The family rightly ask, "Is he becoming demented?" "Is he developing Alzheimer's disease?" Patients with Alzheimer's disease, and the superficially similar Lewy body disease, have mental symptoms of forgetfulness and poor judgement from the beginning, whereas in Parkinson's disease the early symptoms are physical slowness, stiffness or tremor. Although the symptoms of Alzheimer's and Parkinson's overlap and resemble each other, neurologists can usually distinguish these conditions on clinical grounds, sometimes supplemented by brain scans and other tests.

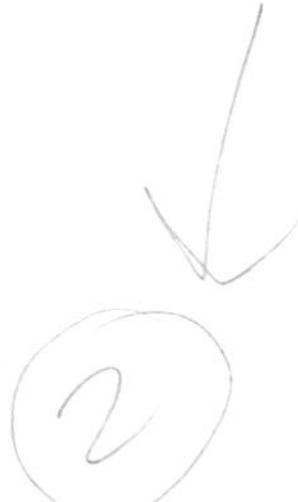

KEY POINTS

- In most cases, an accurate diagnosis is not difficult.
- Parkinson' s disease should not be confused with, and is not caused by, multiple sclerosis or strokes.
- People with Alzheimer's disease have mental symptoms from the beginning, whereas the early symptoms in Parkinson' s disease are physical slowness, stiffness or tremor.

Does Parkinson's disease affect the mind?

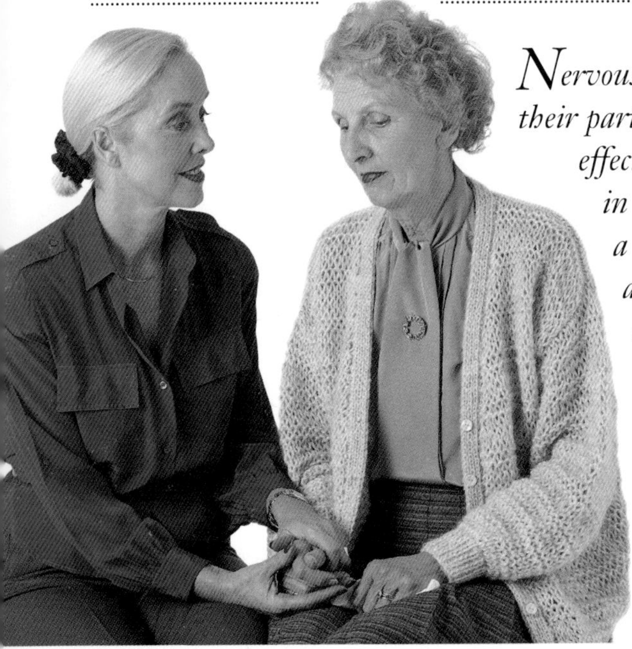

Emotional Effects
Feeling dependent on others may cause anxiety and depression to the Parkinson's disease sufferer.

Nervous and emotional factors play their part in all human disease. The effects of worry and sleeplessness in worsening the pain of even a minor bruise or toothache are as well known as the harmful effects of personal worries on the symptoms of, for example, asthma or a stomach ulcer.

Conversely, if you have a physical illness such as bronchitis, a breast lump, a broken leg or Parkinson's disease, it is not surprising if you feel somewhat anxious, apprehensive or even depressed about it.

The most obvious psychological accompaniments of Parkinson's disease are anxiety or depression caused by the physical symptoms of the disease, and the disability it produces. Tremor and ponderous slow movements are a source of social embarrassment. An abnormal gait, trips and falls, difficulty with speech and voice also embarrass the sufferer. At a very late stage, after many years, the physical handicaps can be severe and restrict many activities; it is no wonder that patients then feel despondent and depressed, particularly about their dependence on others. Fears of future incapacity add to their worries.

DEPRESSION

A depressive illness occurs at some time in about one-third of all Parkinson's disease patients. Depressive illness here means symptoms out of proportion to the underlying cause, or symptoms of such severity that the patient can't cope with them. Depression can occur out of the blue when there is no apparent stress, source of anxiety or physical disability to explain it. This is called endogenous depression. It is of interest that the incidence is higher in people with Parkinson's disease, even before the physical signs are apparent, as compared with the incidence in normal people.

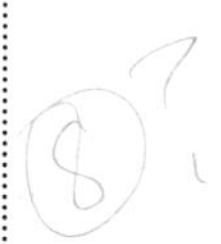

SYMPTOMS OF DEPRESSION

If you have ever been depressed, you will remember the feelings of being miserable, unhappy and low in spirits; you probably also remember the apathy, being devoid of vitality, interests and enthusiasm. Being depressed is quite different from the common complaint of being bored, anxious or just fed up, so commonly expressed by those who are young, disillusioned and unemployed. Depressed patients have to push themselves to make the effort to do everyday tasks – getting dressed, shaving or putting on make up, going out, mixing socially or even having a

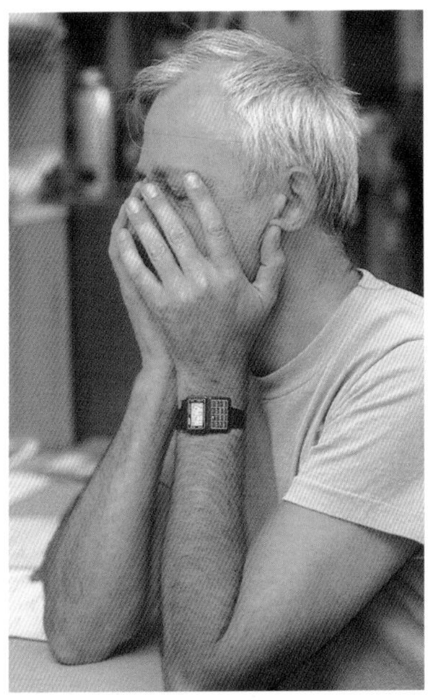

A SENSE OF HOPELESSNESS
A person with depression may feel hopeless and lifeless, and may lack the enthusiasm to do anything constructive. Depression usually responds well to treatment, however.

chat with family or friends. Life seems pointless, hopeless and futile. Sleep is disturbed. Patients go to bed early, just to get away from it all, sleep fitfully until 4 or 5 a.m. and then can sleep no more. Early morning tends to be the worst time, and by evening the blues may have receded a little. These diurnal mood swings are characteristic of the disease.

Physical symptoms of vague pains, headaches, backache, palpitations and often a fear of cancer may dominate their lives, adding to the mental miseries. Feelings of wholly inappropriate guilt are mixed with a sense of inadequacy; if you are depressed, you blame yourself for all your family's misfortunes, and sometimes for all the evils of the world. You will feel periods of restlessness and agitation.

If you feel like this, you need medical attention. Depressed people may commit suicide, but this is fortunately rare in Parkinson's disease.

HOW IS DEPRESSION TREATED?

Symptoms of depression generally respond well to anti-depressant drugs of the tricyclic group (amitriptyline, dothiepin, etc.) but they must be supervised by your GP or specialist. These anti-depressant drugs do not interact with anti-parkinsonian drugs.

Newer anti-depressant drugs are of equal value and include the much-publicised paroxitene (Prozac). Treatment is usually necessary for 6–12 months, sometimes longer. The results are generally good.

CONFUSION

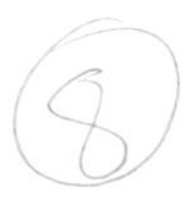

Confusion and hallucinations are uncommon, both in younger patients and in the early stages of the disease. Do not forget that many people over the age of 70 have periods of memory lapses, disorientation and confusion. Deafness and impaired vision can lead to hallucinations in people without Parkinson's disease. When they occur in Parkinson's disease, they may be the result of ageing effects alone, or they may be caused by drugs.

Anti-parkinsonian drugs of all types may cause disorientation, confusion and hallucinations. The most common ones are anticholinergic drugs, for example benzhexol (Artane), orphenadrine (Disipal), benztropine (Cogentin), but bromocriptine (Parlodel) and levodopa drugs (Madopar, Sinemet) can also cause confusional states to arise.

WHAT ARE THE SIGNS OF CONFUSION?

Nightmares and frequent dreams are early warnings of these unpleasant side-effects. In most instances these problems come and go intermittently, but always tend to be more noticeable at night, in strange surroundings, such as hospitals or nursing homes. Disorientation may be related to time, place or person. The patient is bewildered and does not know where her or she is, nor what time of day it is. Recent information is imperfectly registered, so that the patient may deny having had lunch an hour ago, or forget having seen a very recent visitor.

Visual hallucinations consist of seeing things that are not there – seeing people, faces, insects or animals. Auditory hallucinations consist of hearing sounds or voices that are not there – a radio or TV may seem to emit voices, or they may seem to come from inside the patient's head. Sometimes the victim knows they are unreal, having insight into these intrusions, but sometimes he or she may believe them to be real. They can cause distress and agitation.

Confusion may betray itself in peculiar conversation or strange erratic behaviour. Patients may wander off and get lost. They are often inattentive, distractable and memory appears poor because they seem unable to concentrate. Alternatively, they might pour milk into the teapot, put on clothes back to front, attempt to eat puddings with a knife or find themselves unable to tie a knot in their tie, or to use a comb or razor. These latter difficulties are technically called apraxia – the inability to perform skilled movements and sequences when the limbs have normal powers of strength, coordination and sensation.

Drug-related Effects

Although these symptoms may occur in demented patients and are often not totally curable, they may just be a sign of sensitivity to drugs. The doctor will reduce or gradually tail off any possible offending drug and the unpleasant symptoms that the patient has been having will generally disappear.

Obviously, reduction of anti-parkinsonian treatment may lead to an increase in the slowness and rigidity of the disease, but in the end it is easier to handle a sane, but physically slow patient, than a more mobile confused one. A fine balance of drugs, tailored to the individual's needs, will often provide a satisfactory, if not perfect, solution.

DEMENTIA

One of the big worries about Parkinson's disease is that it is known to be associated with dementia – a decline in intellect, memory and the ability to make rational decisions and judgements. This has, without doubt, been overemphasised. Many Parkinsonian patients are not affected in this way and never become demented.

In later life, both Parkinson's disease and Alzheimer's disease, the most frequent cause of dementia, are common. At the age of 70, about 5–10 per cent of the population show some signs of dementia, and about half of these will suffer from Alzheimer's disease. Thus there is a chance that some patients, purely by coincidence, have both parkinsonism and dementia.

The combination is obviously unfortunate and the outlook is considerably worse. Coincidence apart, it is known that about 10–20 per cent of Parkinson's disease patients will develop dementia. If the dementing illness is apparent at the outset, the outlook is worse. If such patients are given levodopa drugs for their parkinsonian symptom, they can tolerate only small doses, and are prone to side-effects, particularly confusional states and hallucinations. In other words, dementia limits the amount of levodopa it is possible to give, and the control of parkinsonian symptoms is less satisfactory for this reason.

The combination of Parkinson's disease and dementia is ultimately disabling. Families will need all the welfare services possible to cope with the patient at home. Ultimately, periods in longer-term hospitals or private nursing homes may be necessary. Research in this very difficult area is active, and there is every hope that progress will be made.

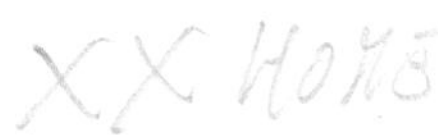

KEY POINTS

- People with Parkinson's disease often feel anxious, apprehensive or even depressed about their illness.
- Medical attention is needed early in depression.
- Confusions and hallucinations may be caused by sensitivity to anti-parkinsonian drugs, or by other unrelated illnesses.
- The combination of Parkinson's disease and dementia makes treatment difficult.

Disability in Parkinson's disease

If you have just been told that you have Parkinson's disease, I expect you will feel gloomy and despondent. You will have visions of a shuffling, bent old person, see yourself in a wheelchair and feel disheartened by the possibility of your family and friends having to look after your every need. These feelings are common, but in many cases they are unjustified by subsequent events.

Being Positive

It is important to understand the illness. and to get it into perspective. Whereas it is true that some patients do end up with severe physical and mental disabilities, many do not. A lot depends on how old you are when the condition is first noticed.

If, for instance, you have been fit and reasonably active and when you are, say, 74 years old you develop a shaking in one hand and a little stiffness and slowness of movement in that arm, we can safely say that your life expectation will not be

Practical Help
Various aids, such as this combination trolley/walking frame, are available to help Parkinson's disease sufferers.

Hoehn and Yahr Scale for Rating Severity of Disability

The Hoehn and Yahr scale recognises five distinct stages of Parkinson's disease.

Stage I
Unilateral disease only.

Stage II
Bilateral mild disease.

Stage III
Bilateral disease with early impairment of postural stability.

Stage IV
Severe disease requiring considerable assistance.

Stage V
Confinement to bed or wheelchair unless aided.

reduced, and that the parkinsonian symptoms are unlikely to cause much disability before you are in your 80s; even then, they may not be serious. Other coincidental illnesses – such as arthritis, bronchitis, heart disease and strokes – are more likely to cause difficulties.

If you are one of those afflicted when unusually young, in your 30s or 40s for example, the rate of deterioration is often slow. Although severe physical problems are eventually likely, you may well have many years of good function and be able to continue with your work and home life. Furthermore, new modifications of treatment have been developing very quickly, with many more drugs available now than there were 10 or 20 years ago. The outlook is likely to continue to improve during the next decade.

DETERIORATION

In general, the course of the illness is a slow one. Sudden deterioration is unlikely unless brought about by other illness, or by use of the wrong drugs. In my experience, and that of others, the disease remains stationary for five or 10 years, or even longer, in as many as perhaps 15–20 per cent of patients, and disabilities are mild and do not increase during this period. Why this should be so, we do not know.

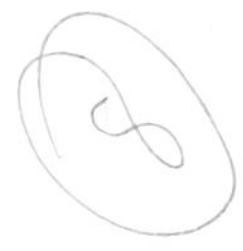

MONITORING TREATMENT

The effects of treatment are vitally important in determining how much trouble the illness causes. The results of treatment are usually most gratifying for several years. In order to assess how effective treatment is, or the stage of the disease at any one time, it is helpful to record the main problems, signs and disabilities. This is done in the consulting room. However, we also have several scales for classifying the stages of the illness. Overall severity is rated on the established, but probably over-simplified, Hoehn and Yahr scale (named after the individuals who developed it).

There are also detailed scales describing problems in walking, feeding, dressing and other activities of daily living (ADL). The lengthy Unified Parkinson's Disease Rating Scale (UPDRS), King's College Hospital Scale and North Western University Disability Scale, are also in common use.

The Webster score (see opposite page) is a simpler scale for assessment, and it takes only 5–10 minutes. It is used by doctors to record slowness of movement (bradykinesia), rigidity, tremor, gait, speech and so on. It comprises 10 items graded 0–3 each, producing scores of 0 (no signs of disability) to a maximum of 30 (most severe). There are two additional useful features: a check on the patient's balance and a check on the ability to get up from a chair.

There are also scales for assessing dyskinesia (jerky, twitching movements). An example of such a scale is

LOSING BALANCE
Poor balance is one of the symptoms assessed on scoring systems. Others include speech, tremor, posture and slowness of movement.

Webster Score for the Assessment of Parkinson's Disease

The Webster's scale is used by practitioners to assess the Parkinson's disease patient's overall pattern of symptoms. It takes about 5–10 minutes to complete the assessment.

STANDARD SYMPTOMS ASSESSED

Each item is graded according to a specific schedule, which is scored 0 (low) to 3 (high):

1. Bradykinesia of hands
2. Rigidity
3. Posture
4. Arm swing
5. Gait
6. Tremor
7. Facial expression
8. Seborrhoea
9. Speech
10. Self-care

ADDITIONAL ITEMS SUGGESTED

(scored 0 to 3, 1 point each):

- Balance
- Rising from chair
- Dyskinesia

MENTAL STATE

(scored 0 to 3)

- Confusion
- Hallucinosis
- Dementia

shown on p.44. You will see that by repeated use of these scales, it is possible to measure the degree of improvement resulting from any form of treatment.

Just as the quality of life has been enhanced by drug treatment, so has the duration of life. Before the levodopa drugs, the life expectancy, after diagnosis was about 12 years. Many Parkinson's disease patients now have a normal life expectancy and death is much more likely to be caused by unrelated, common illnesses that affect the elderly.

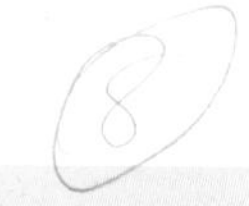

Dyskinesia Scales

These specially designed scales are used by doctors in assessing the severity and duration of a Parkinson's disease patient's dyskinesia, or jerky, twitching movements.

A Duration: The percentage of time when dyskinesia is present during waking hours:

0 = none
1 = 1–25 per cent
2 = 26–50 per cent
3 = 51–75 per cent
4 = 76–100 per cent

B Severity of dyskinesia

0 = noticeable, mild but not disabling
1 = mildly disabling
2 = moderately disabling
3 = severely disabling

NB: Additional scales from 0 to 3 can be made to be used in the assessment of painful dyskinesia and for dystonias.

KEY POINTS

- Not all Parkinson's disease patients end up with severe physical and mental disabilities.
- Specially designed scales are used to assess the severity of disability and the impact of treatment.
- Many patients now have a normal life expectancy.

Medical treatment

Treatment is aimed at abolishing as far as possible the symptoms and disabilities caused by the illness. We do not yet have any drugs that will cure the disease or affect the natural progression. What the available drugs will do is to reverse the symptoms by replacing the essential chemicals, such as dopamine, necessary for the normal transmission of nerve impulses and control of movements.

PART OF THE TREATMENT
Taking drugs is only part of the medical treatment for Parkinson's disease. Although the drugs used cannot prevent brain cell degeneration, they minimise the symptoms of the disorder.

POINTS TO CONSIDER

- Medical treatment should be tailor-made to suit the needs of each individual patient, and will need fine-tuning at intervals over the entire course of the illness. In Parkinson's disease, it is not enough to put the patient on one tablet, three times per day, and leave it at that!
- Treatment should always be governed by symptoms and by disability. For example, at the onset, when the symptoms may be mild and inconspicuous, it is often best to give no drugs at all.
- Correct management of Parkinson's disease means more than drugs alone. Active and positive efforts are

necessary from you and from relatives. Help is also needed from GPs, physiotherapists, occupational therapists and various welfare services at certain times in the disease.

SPECIALIST CARE

In my view, most patients should be referred to a hospital specialist – usually a neurologist – at an early stage in order to confirm the diagnosis, and to obtain advice about the immediate and future prospects of treatment. Patients are seen at intervals to assess their progress and drug treatment. Thereafter, the neurologist will arrange for regular follow-up at intervals that vary from two months to a year. Increasingly, GPs are continuing treatment for patients, but obviously should refer them to the consultant if problems develop.

DRUG TREATMENT

I have already described the deficiency of essential dopamine in the brain and the excess of acetylcholine relative to the dopamine, that occurs in Parkinson's disease. Thus, early treatment consists of drugs called anticholinergics, which diminish acetylcholine and work to restore the balance with dopamine. Many neurologists now leave out this stage, starting drug treatment with small doses of levodopa or a dopamine agonist. Later, amantadine may be introduced; this substance has mild dopamine-releasing properties, boosting dopamine levels; amantadine is weakly anticholinergic and has few side-effects.

Some neurologists introduce dopamine agonists (pergolide or bromocriptine) next, because they cause less jerky, twitching movements (dyskinesia) than

Drugs Used in Parkinson's Disease According to Stage of Disease

The Parkinson's disease patient may be given different drugs during the course of the illness. The drugs prescribed will depend on the severity of symptoms at any particular time.

SYMPTOMS AND DISABILITY	TREATMENT
No disability	No drugs or selegiline
Symptoms a nuisance/ embarrassment	Anticholinergics* and/or selegiline
Stiff and slow despite anticholinergics	Add amantadine or pergolide†
Slow, marked tremor, falls, work in jeopardy	Levodopa given as Madopar or Sinemet
Early dyskinesia or fluctuations	Smaller doses often + pergolide†
Late levodopa failure	Long-acting Madopar or Sinemet + pergolide, or apomorphine injections

* Not in elderly or confused people.
† Pergolide, bromocriptine and lysuride are alternative, similar drugs. Note: combinations of drugs are often used.

levodopa, the drug most often used for established disease. However, within the first 3–4 years, most patients do need a levodopa drug. Levodopa is converted to active dopamine. The old pure form of levodopa has now been replaced by combinations of levodopa with carbidopa (Sinemet), or levodopa with benserazide (Madopar).

Chemical Imbalance in Parkinson's Disease

The levels of acetylcholine and dopamine in the brain are normally balanced. In Parkinson's disease the cells that produce dopamine degenerate, resulting in an insufficient level of dopamine, and relative overactivity of acetylcholine.

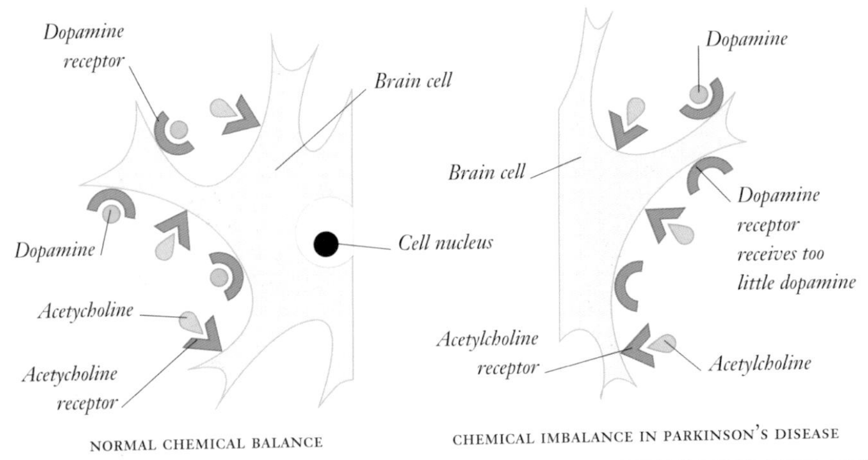

NORMAL CHEMICAL BALANCE

CHEMICAL IMBALANCE IN PARKINSON'S DISEASE

These drugs are the mainstay of drug treatment and more effective than other drugs currently available. Several drugs are available as syrups and elixirs for patients who have difficulty swallowing tablets or capsules. The striking benefits afforded by these drugs may, in some cases, slowly wear off after 5–10 years, but still offer some relief of symptoms. Patients' needs and responses to therapy vary widely, so do not take too literally the dosages or regimens mentioned here.

If the levodopa drugs are not adequate, another group of drugs, called dopamine agonists, may be used. They stimulate the dopamine receptors rather than supply more dopamine. Pergolide, bromocriptine and lysuride are examples of dopamine agonists.

Effect of Drugs Used in Parkinson's Disease

The balance between dopamine and acetylcholine in the brain can be restored by either a drug that blocks the acetylcholine receptors in the brain (an anticholinergic drug), or a dopamine-boosting drug, which increases dopamine activity.

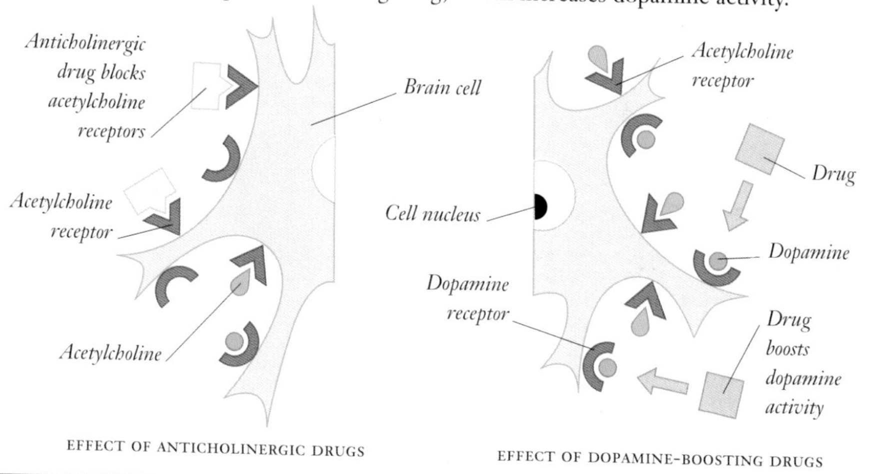

Sometimes, apomorphine is used, but this drug has to be administered by regular injections, rather like a diabetic patient using insulin. It has the great advantage of giving about one hour's (50–90 minutes) benefit starting within 5–10 minutes of the injection; this is useful in helping a sufferer handle a pressing social or business engagement.

Selegiline is itself a weak anti-parkinsonian drug, but it is valuable during the early stages of the disease in order to control symptoms and delay by about one year the introduction of Madopar or Sinemet. Selegiline also reduces the wearing off of the effects of Madopar and Sinemet that occurs in the later stages of the disease (end-of-dose akinesia).

ANTICHOLINERGIC DRUGS

These drugs are valuable for treating early tremor and rigidity, but are not as potent as levodopa in treating slowness, freezing and falls. They are good at controlling salivation and drooling, since they cause a dry mouth. They work well with levodopa drugs, but are generally tailed off gradually in older patients, or if there is any tendency to confusion, hallucination or memory impairment. Symptoms from an enlarged prostate gland, or any liability to glaucoma may be worsened. Anticholinergics are particularly helpful in drug-induced parkinsonian states and in the now rare post-encephalitic

Anticholinergic Drugs

These drugs may be used to treat Parkinson's disease in its early stage, when the symptoms are mild. They are generally used in younger patients who do not have the added complications of the elderly.

DRUG	TRADE NAME	SINGLE DOSE PER TABLET OR CAPSULE	DOSE RANGE PER DAY
Orphenadrine	Disipal Biorphen (syrup/elixir)	50 mg 25 mg/5 ml	100–300 mg
Benzhexol	Artane Broflex (syrup)	2 or 5 mg 5 mg/5 ml	6–15 mg
Benztropine	Cogentin	2 mg	1–4 mg
Procyclidine	Kemadrin Arpicolin (syrup)	5 mg 2.5 mg/5 ml and 5 mg/5 ml	7.5–30 mg

cases. There is little to choose between the various drugs shown in the table in terms of potency or side-effects.

LEVODOPA DRUGS

These are the treatment of choice for moderate and severe Parkinson's disease. Rigidity, slowness, posture and often tremor are improved by levodopa drugs. Their good effects may be less marked in the elderly and in those with long-standing illness, because such patients may be unable to tolerate a dose large enough to control their symptoms. Levodopa is best given as Sinemet or Madopar.

DRUG DOSE

Treatment is started with a small dose, taken with food. This is gradually increased until the smallest dose necessary to produce acceptable control of symptoms and disability is reached.

Levodopa Drugs

Levopoda drugs are usually prescribed when anticholinergic drugs begin to have less effect. They are successful in treating most of the symptoms of moderate to severe Parkinson's disease.

DRUG TABLET	TRADE NAME	SINGLE DOSE PER TABLET OR CAPSULE	LEVADOPA DOSE RANGE PER DAY
Levodopa with Benserazide	Madopar	62.5/125/250 mg	100–800 mg
	Madopar CR	125 mg	100–1200 mg
Levodopa with Carbidopa	Sinemet	110/275 mg	100–800 mg
	Sinemet LS	62.5 mg	100–800 mg
	Sinemet Plus	125 mg	100–800 mg
	Half Sinemet CR	125 mg	100–1200 mg
	Sinemet CR	250 mg	100–1200 mg

Drugs such as Sinemet and Madopar contain a mixture of levodopa and a second drug that concentrates the levodopa in the brain and minimises the side-effects elsewhere in the body.

For example, Sinemet 110 contains levodopa 100 mg plus carbidopa 10 mg; Madopar 250 contains levodopa 200 mg plus benserazide 50 mg.

The best dose is often a compromise between near-total control of all symptoms and side-effects. Many physicians like to keep a little in reserve for possible future needs. Most patients are untroubled by early side-effects, though occasionally nausea, vomiting or fainting are a nuisance: these are easily overcome by dose adjustments and timing.

Side-effects of Levodopa Drugs

Side-effects are divided into those that occur initially and those that appear after some years.

EARLY SIDE-EFFECTS (first few days and weeks):

Nausea and vomiting

Fainting

LATE SIDE-EFFECTS (after 1–3 years):

Wearing off at end of dose:

Dyskinesia and dystonia

'On-off' fluctuations

Mental confusion and hallucinations

SIDE-EFFECTS

After one or two years, some patients develop abnormal jerky, twitching (choreic) or writhing (athetoid) movements, which are called drug-induced dyskinesia. They occur one to three hours after a dose when brain levels of dopamine are at their peak. They affect the mouth, tongue, lips and cheeks and often the neck, limbs and trunk. They more often trouble the patient's husband or wife than the patients themselves, for they are embarrassing and unsightly, rather than disabling. If severe, they can be reduced or abolished by smaller doses of the drugs, which may then need to be given more frequently. The patients with dyskinesia on Sinemet

275, three times a day, may be relieved of it by Sinemet 110 in five or six doses at intervals of two to three hours. The usual response of Parkinson's disease and other kinds of symptomatic parkinsonism to levodopa and anticholinergic drugs is shown in the table on p.55.

The other important unwanted effects are mental disturbances, such as confusion, disorientation and failing memory and concentration. As you grow older, abnormal movements or mental disturbances may make it necessary to reduce the dosage of levodopa.

This may make you much calmer and more contented, but, it is likely to increase your Parkinsonian features – slowness and rigidity, the difficulties in walking, posture and falls. In the end, most families find it easier to handle a patient who is slow, perhaps immobile, but rational than one who is more active, but disorientated and confused.

WEARING-OFF EFFECTS

At a later stage of Parkinson's disease, the duration of action of drugs seems shorter. You may notice wearing off at the end of each dose (end-of-dose akinesia) before the next tablets are due; or you may be aware of wearing off on waking each morning (early morning akinesia) because the last evening's dose has worn off. Slowness, stiffness and freezing are the most troublesome features. Sometimes a single dose seems to fail to work, often an after-lunch dose. This is sometimes caused by proteins in the stomach and intestine, from the preceding meal, interfering with the absorption of the drug into the bloodstream. Modifying the diet may improve this problem.

The recently developed slow-release (controlled-release or CR) preparations are useful in some patients. A single dose in the evening may reduce the difficulties of turning over in bed or getting up to go to the lavatory. It may also control dystonic cramps in the legs and feet, and may give greater mobility on waking, before the first dose of ordinary levodopa is given.

The single dose of a controlled-release preparation at night needs to be used with the usual daytime regimen of ordinary Madopar or Sinemet.

An alternative regimen is to take the CR preparation alone, regularly in the daytime, in place of the usual levodopa drugs; the levels of drug in the blood and brain tend to be lower and are achieved more slowly. The dose needs to be increased by about 50 per cent above the previous levodopa dosage. This produces a smoother and even response of symptoms and shorter periods of immobility in the 'off' phase. However, many patients find that they are never fully active or 'on', and prefer the usual shorter-acting Sinemet or Madopar.

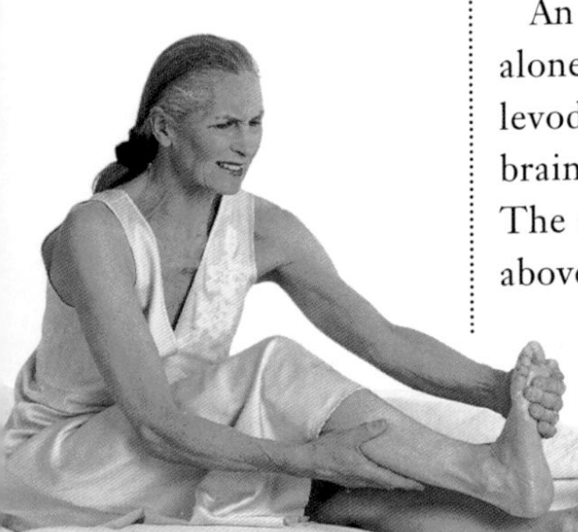

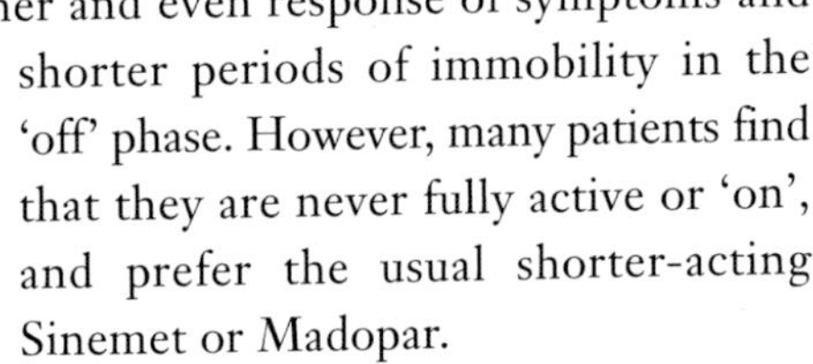

SLOW RELEASE DRUGS *Controlled-release preparations can help to get rid of painful dystonic cramps in some patients.*

'ON-OFF' EPISODES

Later, 'on-off episodes' may develop. The 'on' phase occurs at peak dose and the patient is then mobile and independent, but often has abnormal dyskinetic movements. The 'off' phase consists of sudden freezing, feet sticking to the floor and immobility, sometimes with a feeling of fear and panic. Patients may suddenly switch from 'on' to 'off', and from 'off' to 'on', 'like switching on a light switch'. This is disconcerting, and can sometimes mistakenly be thought to be nervous

How Parkinson's Disease Responds to Drugs

This table shows the usual response of Parkinson's disease and other kinds of symptomatic parkinsonism to levodopa and anticholinergic drugs.

CONDITION	LEVODOPA	ANTICHOLINERGIC DRUGS
Parkinson's disease	●●●	●●
Drug-induced parkinsonism	●●	●●
Multi-system atrophies, including progressive supranuclear palsy	+/-	+/-
Other causes of parkinsonism	+/-	+/-

Key ●●● usually very good ●● moderate +/- variable response

or psychologically caused. Smaller, more frequent doses may ease this difficult problem.

A related problem is painful cramp-like twisting of the ankle and toes that occurs often at the end of the dose, just before the next dose is due, or sometimes at night. This is called drug-induced dystonia.

You will appreciate that all these drug manipulations require patience and skill both from patient and physician. It is often necessary to admit such patients to hospital for specialised care, frequent checks and ratings of symptoms, side-effects and dosage in order to achieve the fine-tuning for optimal performance. This may take one or two weeks.

DOPAMINE AGONISTS

It is fashionable to introduce these drugs at an early stage, before levodopa, because they cause less dyskinesia than levodopa, and, it is thought that they may delay the appearance of levodopa dyskinesias and fluctuations. Another use is to introduce a dopamine agonist when dyskinesia, mental side-effects or 'on-off' fluctuations develop as they stimulate or excite the dopamine receptors into greater activity.

Pergolide, bromocriptine and lysuride are similar dopamine-agonist drugs. Ropinirole has a similar effect and is of about the same strength as levodopa. When used with levodopa, it reduces the wearing off time and may allow a reduction in levodopa dose. Patients with severe vascular, kidney or liver disease, or those pregnant or breast-feeding should not generally take this group of drugs. They are started in small doses and slowly increased every week or so until benefit is apparent without undue side-effects. It may take 2–3 months to find the best stable dose. When taken in combination with Sinemet or Madopar, it may be possible to reduce the levodopa dose by about 25 per cent when the benefit begins.

SIDE-EFFECTS

Dopamine agonists are strong drugs, which reduce all the symptoms of Parkinson's disease, but their side-effects can be prohibitive. They cause more severe psychiatric complications of confusion, delusions and frank aggressive behaviour in a number of patients. These are usually reversible on reducing the dose, but often it is necessary to stop the drug. These psychiatric complications are especially likely in the over 70s and in those with previous confusion or dementia. Dopamine agonists can also

Dopamine Agonists

This chart lists the commonly used dopamine agonists, together with their trade names and typical dosages. Their effect is to stimulate activity of the dopamine receptors.

DRUG	TRADE NAME	SINGLE DOSE	DOSE PER DAY
Bromocriptine	Parlodel	1, 2.5, 5, 10 mg	20–100 mg
Lysuride	Revanil	200 µg*	600–5,000 µg
Pergolide	Celance	50, 250, 1000 µg	750–4,000 µg
Apomorphine	Britaject	10 mg in 2 ml ampoule	3–30 mg
Cabergoline	Cabaser	1, 2, 4 mg	2–6mg
Ropinirole	Requip	0.25, 1, 2, 5 mg	3–9 mg

*Note: 1,000 micrograms (µg) = 1 milligram (mg)

aggravate stomach ulcers and arterial disease in the legs. In general, they should not be given to older patients, and should always be supervised by a specialist.

APOMORPHINE

This is an old drug that has found a new use. It, too, is a dopamine agonist, but it has to be given by a pump or by injections subcutaneously (under the skin) in the lower abdomen or outer thigh, which many patients or relatives can be taught to give. It causes vomiting unless each dose is preceded by domperidone, a potent anti-vomiting drug taken by mouth.

Apomorphine injections can be helpful, giving about one hour's (50–90 minutes) almost certain benefit starting within 5–10 minutes of the injection. This is useful if you have an important social or business engagement. The injections can be repeated two or three times each day, under specialist advice. Dyskinesia can result if the dose is too high, and the correct dose for you has to be found by trial and error, always starting with a small dose.

Of many new groups of drugs being assessed entacopone works by inhibiting an enzyme (catechol-O-methyltransferase) that breaks down levodopa and hence prolongs its duration of action. Tolcapone has been withdrawn because of occasional serious side-effects. Entacapone requires further clinical experience to assess its effectiveness and safety. This group of drugs improves motor function, that is, strength and coordinated movements, and the duration of the 'on' phase, and reduces the levopoda dosage. Lazabemide (RO19-6327) is a short-acting, selective inhibitor of monoamine oxidase-B type, similar to selegiline. A significant improvement in the activities of daily living has been found after four weeks of lazabemide treatment, and side-effects appear minimal.

SELEGILINE (ELDEPRYL)

This is a weak anti-parkinsonian drug, but it slightly strengthens the effects of levodopa drugs, and it may reduce the 'on-off' swings, especially the immobility in the 'off' phase. It is best given early in the illness, and is useful because it controls most of the early symptoms for one or two years.

The early reports that selegiline had a protective effect, slowing down the disease, have sadly proved to be untrue. A single dose of 10 mg each morning is well tolerated, and side-effects are not common. One group of UK researchers has found a small increased mortality rate and a tendency to fainting attacks (syncope) in some patients treated with selegiline, though most published series do not show any such effects. No reason for this has been shown and since a causal link is not yet established most physicians continue to use the drug in standard dosage.

DRUG HOLIDAYS

In resistant cases with random 'on-off' swings and poor control of parkinsonian symptoms, drug holidays have been tried. The aim is that, by withdrawal of drugs, an attempt is made to rest or to reset the dopamine receptors that have been overdriven by levodopa and other drugs, and to rid the brain of theoretical toxic byproducts of these drugs. This is all unproven speculation and, in practice, benefits only sufferers who are plainly overdosed.

Restabilisation, in hospital, is then necessary with hourly recording charts of Parkinsonian signs, disability, mental performance and side-effects. These observations usually reveal the problem, and then we often stop inessential or weak acting drugs and those medications

Other Drugs

Typical doses of two other drugs commonly used to treat Parkinson's disease are shown in this chart.

DRUG	TRADE NAME	DOSE	DOSE PER DAY
Amantadine	Symmetrel	100 mg	200 mg
Selegiline	Eldepryl Eldepryl syrup	10 mg 10 mg/5 ml	5-10 mg

thought to be unnecessary for coincidental ailments. The dose of levodopa is reduced by 50–75 per cent and, as side-effects disappear, drugs are reintroduced gradually until the smallest effective dose is found. Simplification is the hallmark of effective treatment.

In difficult cases, it is sometimes helpful to apply an apomorphine or levodopa test dose. A single high dose is given after a 24-hour period of drug withdrawal, and the effects give a good indication of whether or not the dopamine receptors are still responsive. If they are not, there is plainly no sense in persisting with dopaminergic drugs. The test gives important information that predicts future responses to treatment. A single dose of 250 mg Madopar or an injection of 2–10 mg apomorphine will demonstrate dopamine responsiveness by showing improvement of at least 20 per cent in one of the standard rating scales I discussed earlier.

DRUG WARNINGS

Certain drugs should not be used in Parkinson's disease. I have mentioned the major phenothiazine tranquillisers and antipsychotic drugs (neuroleptics). These drugs may also be suggested for nausea or for dizzy attacks, but should seldom be used in Parkinson's disease. Monoamine oxidase inhibitors used for depression are not allowed, but tricyclic antidepressants are in order. Patients with certain types of glaucoma or skin melanoma should not take levodopa drugs.

Vitamin B6 (pyridoxine), present in multi-vitamin capsules and medicines, and used for premenstrual tension, blocks the action of levodopa, but there is no interaction if given with Sinemet or Madopar. If in doubt, you should always consult your doctor.

GENE THERAPY

In addition to new drugs, there are other new approaches to treatment. Gene therapy holds considerable potential for the treatment of central nervous system disease. The introduction of functional genes into the brain of patients with Parkinson's disease may prove useful as a means to replace a defective gene. It aims to introduce a protein, which can protect against cell damage or restore the workings of a damaged cell, or permit the physiological delivery of a deficient neurotransmitter. The strategies for gene therapy techniques have expanded beyond the classical dopamine replacement, toward the use of factors that induce nerve cell growth (neurotrophic factors) in enhancing cell function or preventing cell death.

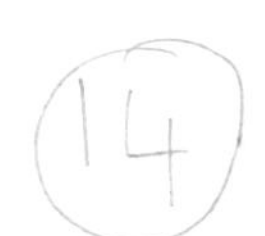

KEY POINTS

- Drug treatment reverses the symptoms of Parkinson's by replacing the essential chemicals necessary for normal transmission of nerve impulses and control of movements.
- Drugs are chosen to match the stage of the disease and need adjustments at intervals throughout the illness.
- Combinations of levodopa with carbidopa (Sinemet) or with benserazide (Madopar) are the most effective drugs.
- Unwanted side-effects can be reduced or abolished by altering the drug dose and timing.
- When wearing-off effects of drugs are troublesome, the recently developed slow-release (controlled release or CR) preparations are useful in a few patients.
- Dopamine agonists should not be given to older patients and should always be supervised by a specialist.

Surgery for Parkinson's disease

Surgery consists of either destruction of tiny parts of the brain (stereotactic surgery) or transplantation of dopamine-producing tissue into the brain.

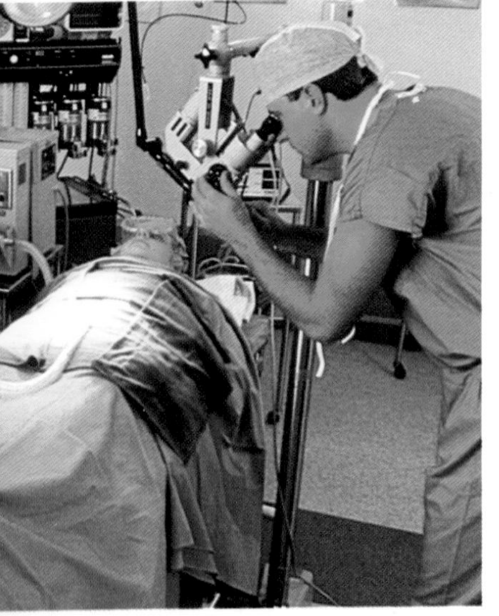

SURGICAL TREATMENT
Although few operations are carried out at present. research into new surgical treatments for Parkinson's disease is continuing.

STEREOTACTIC SURGERY

Surgical treatment for Parkinson's disease is rarely recommended. Thirty years ago there was a vogue for placing tiny destructive lesions in the basal ganglia by means of a stereotactic apparatus that permitted very accurate placement of the lesion. This technique was fairly effective in controlling tremor and rigidity – if it was one-sided. Stereotactic surgery is of no benefit in correcting the facial expression, weak voice, slowness of movement, stooped posture and tendency to fall. Indeed, sometimes these symptoms are made worse.

Stereotactic surgery is still used, especially in Japan, for early one-sided tremor and rigidity, if they fail to respond to other measures. In most specialised centres in the UK and the USA, however, it is seldom used because levodopa drugs, despite their shortcomings, have, in general, proved so effective. Occasional patients may benefit from such operations if their main problem is one-sided shaking and rigidity that is uncontrollable by drug treatment. The decision requires expert neurological advice. New techniques are being developed, but require time before their benefits and risks can be fully assessed. Stereotactic Gamma thalamotomy has met with some success, reducing rigidity and also tremor in otherwise resistant cases.

NIGRAL TRANSPLANTS

In 1981 in Sweden, the first attempts were made to transplant the patient's own adrenal medulla (autografts) into the caudate nucleus, a part of the basal ganglia involved in the transmission of dopamine. The adrenal medulla is rich in amines, including dopamine. The hope was that this would provide an added source of natural dopamine. Results in early patients were disappointing, and any doubtful benefit wore off quickly. This work did, however, show that the surgery was possible, that the adrenal tissue took on its new blood supply and, to some extent, formed new nerve connections in the receptor site.

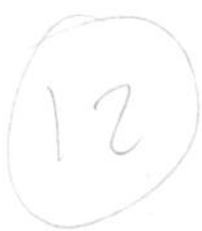

More publicity was given to the extension of this work in younger patients in Mexico. This was not a controlled study, and the florid publicity in the national press caused more than a little sceptical criticism amongst neuroscientists worldwide. Isolated reports of similar procedures in North America have confirmed the correctness of this cautious reception. Subsequent operations transplanting the adrenal medulla have shown variable and slight benefits. Adrenal grafts survive poorly following implantation, but they are capable of inducing sprouting of nerve fibres in the host's caudate nucleus. This approach has been abandoned.

FETAL TISSUE TRANSPLANT

Other methods have been attempted, notably the transplantation of substantia nigra from human fetuses. This area is the main focus of loss of dopamine stores in human Parkinson's disease, so it makes good sense to replace it with the same tissue.

PROBLEMS WITH SURGERY

The number of such operations is still small, largely because it requires major surgery at centres with specialised experience; there are ethical problems in obtaining and using fetal donor tissue, and the long-term benefits are not yet known. The number of patients likely to benefit from current techniques is small.

Strict scientific control comparing operated against non-operated cases of similar age, sex and severity of illness is essential before we can say that the operation is valuable in certain types or stages of the disease, or, conversely, of no benefit to any patient. However, it is encouraging that robust survival of fetal nigral implants can be achieved within the human brain; these can give a new nerve supply to the damaged nerve cells in the basal ganglia.

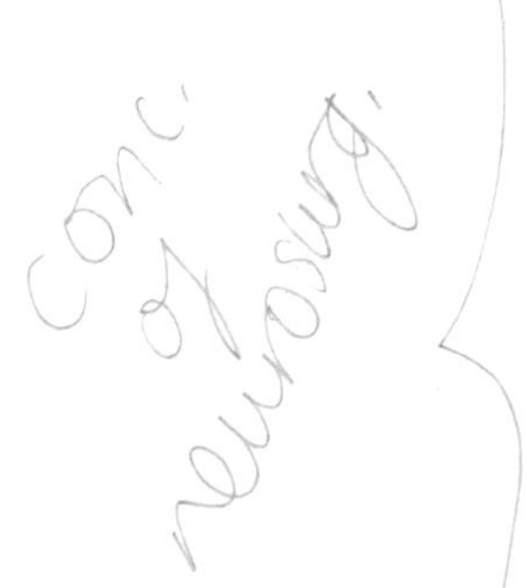

For the present, these techniques continually advance, but must be viewed with cautious optimism. It is not known whether transplantation alters the progression or outcome of Parkinson's disease. It is not known whether any such benefit will be lasting. And it is not known whether those agent(s) that primarily cause the disease will also destroy the graft. We must also remember that Parkinson's disease reflects a disorder not only of dopamine transmission, but of many other neurotransmitters that may not be replaced by the grafts, even if the grafts work. These techniques hold out promise, but we do not know if they will have a lasting place in the treatment of a small minority of patients. Meanwhile, no patient should feel deprived of an implant until much more research has been completed.

KEY POINTS

- Stereotactic surgery can occasionally be beneficial for one-sided shaking and rigidity uncontrollable by drug treatment.
- Attempts to transplant dopamine-rich fetal tissue into the brains of patients with Parkinson's disease need to be repeated under strictly controlled conditions before the value of such surgery can be judged.

General management

Drug treatment is the most important single measure in reversing the symptoms and disabilities of Parkinson's disease, but there is far more to the treatment of the patient than just the administration of drugs.

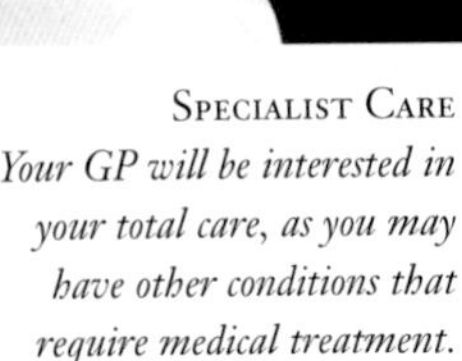

Specialist Care
Your GP will be interested in your total care, as you may have other conditions that require medical treatment.

Many of the problems that are faced by patients are not caused by Parkinson's disease itself, but by the coincidental accompanying conditions from which many people suffer, and which may need separate medical attention. Some patients are diabetic, some have high blood pressure, some asthma, some heart disease or bronchitis, and many have arthritis. The care of the whole patient is therefore an essential approach from your doctor – GP or specialist.

Identifying the Problems

Certain problems occur commonly in Parkinson's disease and the first step is to identify them. Then, we must outline means of helping to correct them. Here are some common problems in movement that you may have noticed, and there are many more:

- Walking slowly.
- Walking with short, shuffling steps.
- Walking through doorways, causing you to stop or hesitate.
- Freezing of feet to the floor.
- Turning in a narrow space without falling.
- Swinging the arms automatically when walking.
- Getting out of a chair.
- Standing straight instead of hunched forwards.
- Turning over in bed.
- Getting on and off a toilet.
- Using the hands with fine manipulations, dressing and undressing.
- Writing smaller, shaky and spidery.
- Using a screwdriver.
- Sewing on buttons or crocheting.

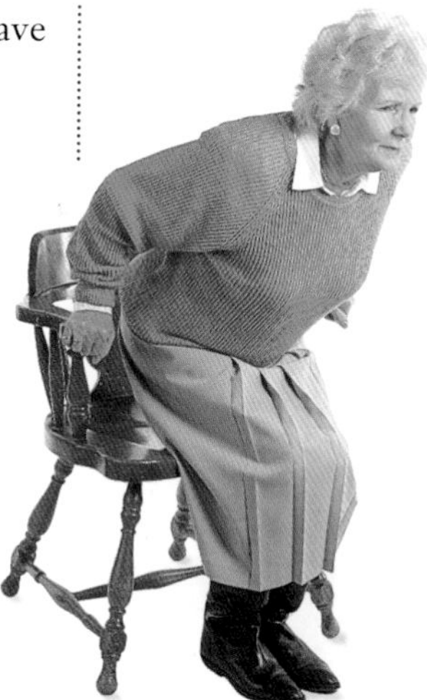

MOBILITY PROBLEMS
Simple physical movements, such as getting out of a chair, may become increasingly difficult for the Parkinson's disease sufferer as physical disabilities hinder action.

PHYSIOTHERAPY

Physiotherapy has specific benefits for specific problems; it also has a generally beneficial effect in boosting morale, in persuading the patient that something active is being done and that he or she is playing an active part in the treatment. The motivation, personality and the attitude of both patient and therapist have a marked influence on the general benefits obtained. Bad habits are better eradicated early than late. In advanced illness, motivation may be poor, memory and concentration impaired and effective cooperation may be impossible.

Assessment is the first step. This includes:

- Physical disabilities.
- Learning capacity and mental state.

- Home circumstances.
- The availability of able-bodied friends and family to continue to practice any instructions.

EXERCISES

Exercises and activity are important, as they mobilise joints and muscles, lessen stiffness and improve posture. They aim to:

- Correct abnormal gait.
- Correct bad posture.
- Prevent or minimise stiffness and contractures of the joints.
- Improve use and facilities of the limbs.
- Provide a regimen that can be used at home by the patient.

Regular exercise is beneficial whenever disabilities permit. It helps to maintain your muscle tone and strength, and helps to prevent contractures and stiffening. Walking is one of the most valuable exercises. Most people in the early stages of Parkinson's disease can walk a mile or two each day, sometimes much more. A conscious effort should be made to keep the back straight, the shoulders back and the head upright, and to take slow, long strides. Even more severely affected people can often walk 300 or 400 yards, and perhaps repeat this once or twice every day. Slippery surfaces, snow, ice and wet leaves should obviously be avoided.

The physiotherapist will concentrate on teaching you to sit straight, often in a high upright chair, aided by a cushion in the back. She or he will show you how to concentrate on striking the heel down when walking, how to improve moving from sitting to standing, by pulling your heels in under the front edge of the chair and throwing your weight forwards as you get up. Standing in front of a long mirror may help you to see and correct any stoop or bent posture of the neck and trunk.

Self-motivation

Constant repetition and practice are necessary at home, especially when the therapist is no longer badgering you; there is no substitute for 'do it yourself'! Exercises may be made easier and more rhythmical if performed to music on a cassette, CD or radio. Visits to out-patient therapy may be helpful and encouragement may be obtained by group exercises. Therapeutic holidays, including vigorous activity, can also be arranged (see Useful addresses p.77).

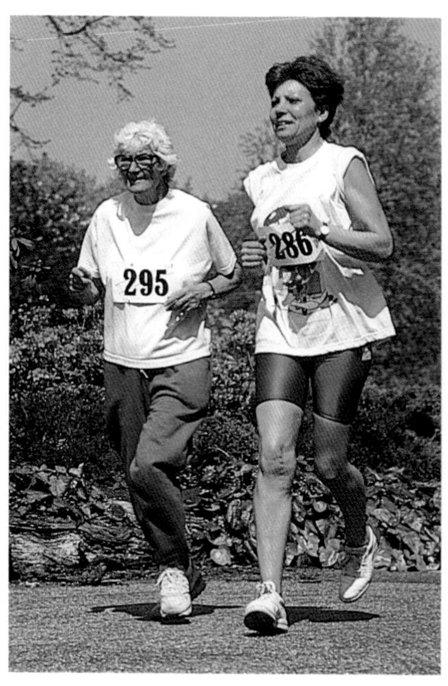

Vigorous Exercise
With regular practice, some patients find themselves able to undertake quite strenuous exercise, and specially tailored therapeutic holidays are available.

Occupational Therapy

A wide range of home aids is available, many of which should be available on the NHS, although some may need to be purchased privately. A home visit by an occupational therapist is invaluable, and he or she will usually prepare a report for the hospital consultant describing specific problems, the need for gadgets, hand rails, high seats and other provisions. Wide handles on cutlery, antislip kitchen surfaces, lever arms on taps, raised working surfaces in the kitchen and greenhouse, Velcro fasteners to garments and shoes, are examples of the ways in which you can make easier your activities and independence.

APPLIANCES

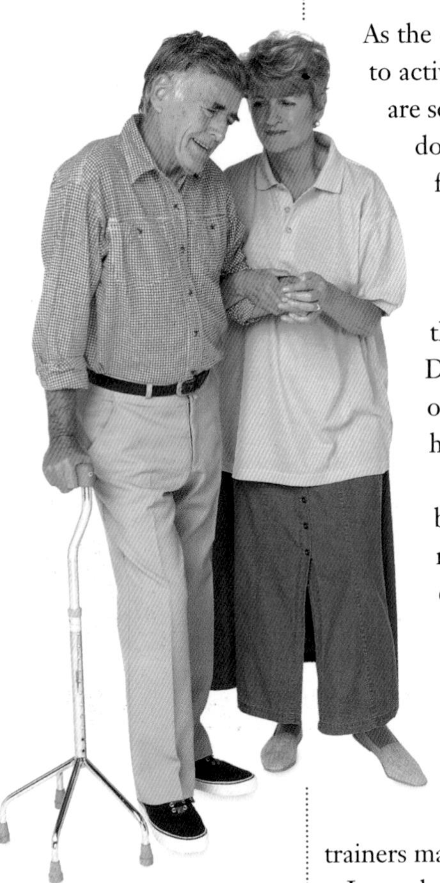

INCREASING MOBILITY
Walking aids, such as the one shown here, can help to promote independence in the Parkinson's disease patient.

As the disease progresses, some patients require aids to activity. Walking sticks add to your stability and are socially unobtrusive. A tripod held in one hand does the same thing on a wider base. Zimmer frames are not recommended, except as a short-term measure when mobilising after injury or operation in hospital. They break the natural rhythm of walking. If, however, they are fitted with wheels, they are valuable. Delta frames with two 'legs' and a front wheel, or a rotator with two legs and two wheels are helpful. Brakes add to your sense of security.

Individual exercises are aimed to help balance, lengthen your stride and perhaps relieve the pain of a frozen shoulder – a common complication.

Manual dexterity may be improved by practice with blocks, jigsaws and certain games. Grab rails fitted near your bed, in the lavatory and bathroom are helpful. Buttons and zips can be replaced by Velcro fasteners. Casual or elastic sided shoes or trainers may be much easier than lace-up shoes.

Large-handled knives, forks and spoons, stick-on plates and egg cups can save spills. Many of these can be supplied or recommended by the physiotherapist or occupational therapist. The Welfare Department of the Parkinson's Disease Society is also able to advise.

It is of enormous advantage if there is good liaison between the hospital-based physiotherapist, occupational therapist, the social worker and the ward team. They will meet to discuss plans and joint assessments when patients are admitted to the ward, and will continue supervision, where possible, after you go home. They will also link up with the GP and district welfare services.

Speech Therapy

Many patients are embarrassed and frustrated by their speech. You may find that you speak quietly, are unable to shout and that friends are always asking you to repeat yourself, or to speak up. Speech may be slurred and hesitant with lack of variation in pitch and volume of the voice. Assessment by a speech therapist will examine the way you breathe, move your lips, tongue and jaw in the formation of speech – all elements that we do unconsciously or automatically.

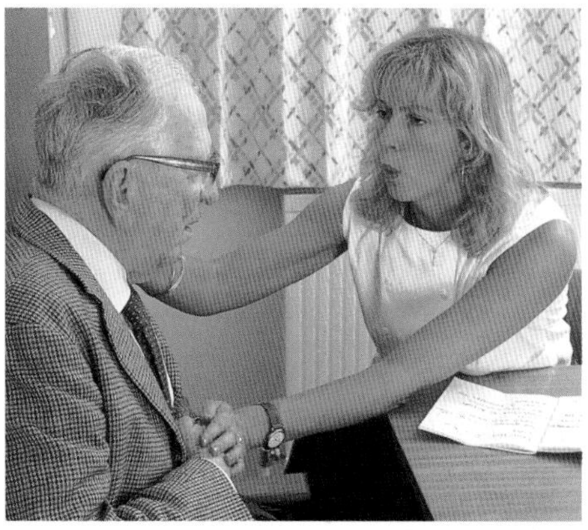

Improving Speech
Speech therapy can give some help in retraining the voice and speech of a patient, but improvements are limited.

In Parkinson's disease, the voice box (larynx) no longer works properly, producing a monotonous pitch, lack of volume control and lack of stress of certain sounds. Your voice may sound hoarse, quiet and monotonous. Speech therapy may use audio feedback in which you hear your own speech after a measured latent interval; this can modify and improve the voice and speech output. This and other manoeuvres can, to a modest extent, help to retrain the voice and speech, but dramatic improvements are not common.

Communication Aids

Aids to communication include 'Edu-Com Scanning', a device to point to a word or picture showing your intention and meaning. 'Micro-writer' links a TV, printer or speech synthesiser and can be of occasional help to

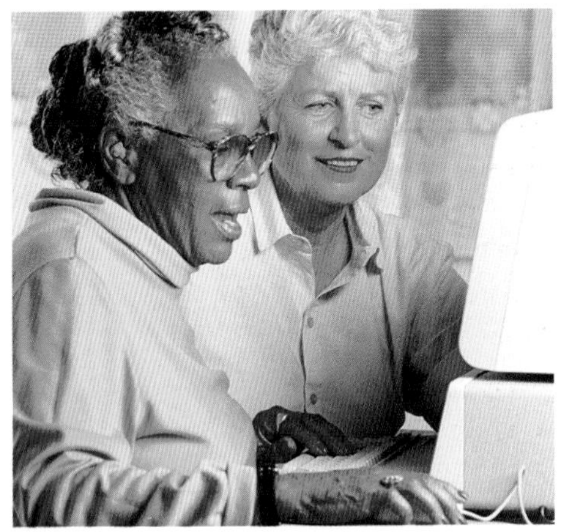

WRITING AID
For patients who find writing difficult, a small home computer may prove an invaluable ally.

patients when speech training is unsuccessful. The use of a personal computer (PC) may help you to write letters and perform business activities and attend to your finances from home. Modern programmes are fairly easy to learn if you are a newcomer to this technological world, and there is a wide range of recreational games and educational material that may occupy and expand your interests.

DIET

Patients with Parkinson's disease require no special diets, but should have a balanced enjoyable diet with fresh meat, fish, fruit and vegetables, like everyone else. Sometimes, a dose of Madopar or Sinemet does not work, particularly with an after-lunch dose. This may occur because proteins in the stomach and intestine from the preceding meal can interfere with the absorption of the drug into the bloodstream. Your specialist may advise you to have a low-protein lunch with small amounts of meat, fish, poultry, eggs or cheese, but to include these foods in the main evening meal, after which you may not wish to be as active as during the day.

GENERAL OBSERVATIONS

With the help of your GP you should obtain up-to-date medical support and supervision of your drug and physical treatment, and advice about any possible side-effects. More specialised guidance is available from consultants in clinics, who should supervise most patients, where staffing levels and facilities permit. The welfare services and hospital units also provide support from physiotherapists, occupational therapists and social workers when the need arises, but currently, the provision and quality of support is variable.

Activity throughout the illness is the keynote. Do as much as you can, but be sensible and do not over-do it to the point of exhaustion. Three walks of 400 yards each are at least as beneficial as one of 1,200 yards. You will also have to make certain adjustments to your lifestyle, but these are usually obvious, and changes are gradual, so you have plenty of time to make these alterations. You may have to allow a little longer to get dressed or go to work, or to plan and pack for holidays or journeys. It may take two goes to mow the lawn instead of one. Try not to let this irritate you; a little planning, allowing more time, will make most tasks possible.

Do not get fanatical about crack-pot schemes you read about, or about gossip you hear. A lot of money can be wasted on charlatan remedies, health foods, acupuncture, osteopathy and so forth. Medical opinion has no rooted objections to these therapies, but does not use them unless they have been carefully and scientifically tested, so that it is clear if they are of benefit or not.

Conclusions

Although there has been considerable progress in the last few years, Parkinson's disease remains something of an enigma. We know that there is degeneration of certain small, but vital, areas of the brain, but it is not just a condition caused by ageing. Its effects are complex, but the main one is a lack of an essential chemical transmitter, dopamine, which can be effectively replaced by modern drug treatment. This permits a full and active life for many years.

Medical and social research is funded on a large scale by the Parkinson's Disease Society and by other organisations. As a result, hardly a year goes by without some important addition to knowledge – additions that are of practical importance to each and every sufferer from the disease.

All new discoveries require careful scientific scrutiny before they can be accepted as valid. There are many avenues of progress under investigation.

Although we are dealing with a slowly progressing illness in most cases, you should remember that most patients have a normal life-span, which includes many years of activity and enjoyment. Sufferers from Parkinson's disease can face the future with measured optimism.

KEY POINTS

- An exercise programme can be developed with the help of a physiotherapist.
- Many aids are available to encourage independence in the home.
- Speech may be improved by working with a speech therapist.
- Patients should eat a healthy, balanced diet, but no special diets are necessary.

Questions and answers

What causes Parkinson's disease?
We do not know the cause. Investigations have sought environmental factors such as contaminants of food, water and air and exposure to poisonous chemicals at work, but have failed to produce an answer. Although there is a weak hereditary factor, it is not the cause, but may make certain people more susceptible to unidentified substances, to which we may be exposed.

I have been under a lot of stress. Could that be the cause?
No. Stress and tension may cause a temporary worsening of symptoms, but they do not cause the disease. Depression is a common problem in Parkinson's disease, and may reduce your general efficiency, drive and ability to cope. It is generally much improved by anti-depressant drugs.

Will I pass it on to my children or grandchildren?
Although there is a slightly higher incidence of perhaps one in 20 cases in close relatives, Parkinson's disease is not an inherited disease.

I have heard that selegiline (Eldepryl) will slow down the disease. Should I take it?
Trials in the USA have now shown that selegiline does not affect the disease process in the brain and has no effect in reducing the rate of progression. It is, nonetheless, useful early in the illness and acts by relieving early symptoms, thereby delaying the time when it is necessary to start levodopa drugs. Side-effects are infrequent and mild.

Is there any advantage in delaying the start of levodopa drugs?
Because the benefit of levodopa drugs tends to fade after 5–10 years, it is generally thought sensible not to start them too soon, i.e., before symptoms are of more than nuisance value, and are beginning to interfere with work and leisure.

There is no advantage in delaying once this time is reached, and the benefits are usually obvious and will improve your quality of life.

What will be the effects of levodopa, and will it have side-effects?
Within a month or so, stiffness, slowness of movements, walking difficulties and posture start to improve. Shaking does not always disappear, but may be reduced. Benefit continues to increase as the fine tuning of dose and timing are carefully monitored. A few patients have sickness or faintness in the first few weeks, but taking tablets on a full stomach, and starting with small doses that are increased slowly will allow them to cope with this. Abnormal movements, fluctuations in effects – before and after each dose, and mental problems can develop later in the illness, but adjustments of drugs and dosage often improve or abolish these symptoms.

I have taken dopamine (Madopar) for two years. Why am I now getting these funny twitching movements?
These are probably dyskinesias or dystonias caused by a slight over-spill or excess of drug on the sensitive receptors in the brain. They usually occur some 30–60 minutes after each dose, and last for a few minutes. Your doctor may advise a slight reduction in dose, given at shorter intervals. A controlled release (CR) preparation helps some patients.

Why is it taking so long for the tablets to work, and why do they wear off so quickly?
After a few years the body does not absorb or distribute levodopa as efficiently, and the dopamine receptors do not respond quite so effectively, as at the start of treatment. Alteration by your physician of the dose and frequency often overcomes this problem.

I find that I cannot concentrate or remember things as I used to. Is Parkinson's disease responsible?
Memory and concentration often diminish with normal ageing, irrespective of Parkinson's disease. If you have become depressed, this can also affect concentration and memory, and often improves with simplification of, or additional, drug therapy. Only a small percentage of Parkinson's disease sufferers become demented.

Am I likely to benefit from a transplant?
Adrenal transplants are now thought to be largely ineffective. Fetal transplants are, for the time being, in the experimental stage. They have been shown to be feasible, but their value is not yet established. Meanwhile, no patient should feel deprived of an implant until we have far more information.

Useful addresses and publications

Help and Information

Parkinson's Disease Society
215 Vauxhall Bridge Road,
London SW1V 1EJ
Telephone: (0171) 931 8080.

Citizens Advice Bureau
For local information and up-to-date addresses. see your local telephone directory.

Disabled Living Foundation
Visits by appointment only for advice about equipment and appliances.
380-384 Harrow Road,
London W9 2HU
Telephone: (0171) 289 6111.

Publications

Help for Handicapped People
A DHSS booklet available from the Parkinson's Disease Society or your local social security office.

Coping with Disablement
Published by the Consumers' Association,
2 Marylebone Road,
London NW1 4DF.

Holidays for the Physically Handicapped
From the Central Council for the Disabled,
34 Eccleston Square,
London SW1V 1PE.

Index

Acknowledgements

PUBLISHER'S ACKNOWLEDGEMENTS
Dorling Kindersley would like to thank the following for their help and participation in this project:

Production Controller Michelle Thomas; **Consultancy** Dr. Sue Davidson; **Indexing** Indexing Specialists, Hove; **Administration** Christopher Gordon.

Organisations St. John's Ambulance, St. Andrew's Ambulance Organisation, British Red Cross.

Illustrations (p.61) ©Philip Wilson.

Picture Research Angela Anderson; **Picture Librarian** Charlotte Oster.

PICTURE CREDITS
The publisher would like to thank the following for their kind permission to reproduce their photographs. Every effort has been made to trace the copyright holders. Dorling Kindersley apologises for any unintentional omissions and would be pleased, in any such cases, to add an acknowledgement in future editions.

Sally & Richard Greenhill Photo Library p.34, pp.69; **Robert Harding** p. 7, p.72 (Patrick Ramsey); **Science Photo Library** p.18 (Gary Watson), p.26 (Tirot/BSIP), p.62 (Stevie Grand), p.71 (Hattie Young).